Curbside
Consultation
in Endoscopy

49 Clinical Questions

Curbside Consultation in Gastroenterology
SERIES

SERIES EDITOR, FRANCIS A. FARRAYE

Curbside Consultation

in Endoscopy

49 Clinical Questions

Joseph Leung, MD, FRCP, FACP, FACG, FASGE
Chief of Gastroenterology
Veterans Affairs Northern California Health Care System
Mr. & Mrs. C.W. Law Professor of Medicine
University of California, Davis School of Medicine
Sacramento, CA

and

Simon Lo, MD
Director, Pancreatic and Biliary Diseases Program
Director, GI Endoscopy
Cedars-Sinai Medical Center
Los Angeles, CA

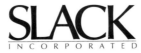

SLACK
INCORPORATED

Delivering the best in health care information and education worldwide

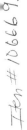

Published by: SLACK Incorporated
                       6900 Grove Road
                       Thorofare, NJ 08086 USA
                       Telephone: 856-848-1000
                       Fax: 856-853-5991
                       www.slackbooks.com

Contact SLACK Incorporated for more information about other books in this field or about the availability of our books from distributors outside the United States.

Library of Congress Cataloging-in-Publication Data

Curbside consultation in endoscopy : 49 clinical questions / [edited by] Joseph Leung and Simon Lo.
      p. ; cm. -- (Curbside consultation in gastroenterology series)
  Includes bibliographical references and index.
  ISBN-13: 978-1-55642-817-3 (alk. paper)
  ISBN-10: 1-55642-817-0 (alk. paper)
  1. Endoscopy--Miscellanea. I. Leung, J. W. C. II. Lo, Simon. III. Series: Curbside consultation in gastroenterology.
  [DNLM: 1. Endoscopy, Digestive System--methods. 2. Digestive System Diseases--diagnosis. 3. Digestive System Diseases--therapy. WI 141 C975 2008]
  RC78.7.E5C87 2008
  616.07'545--dc22
                              2008034676

For permission to reprint material in another publication, contact SLACK Incorporated. Authorization to photocopy items for internal, personal, or academic use is granted by SLACK Incorporated provided that the appropriate fee is paid directly to Copyright Clearance Center. Prior to photocopying items, please contact the Copyright Clearance Center at 222 Rosewood Drive, Danvers, MA 01923 USA; phone: 978-750-8400; website: www.copyright.com; email: info@copyright.com

Printed in the United States of America.

Last digit is print number: 10   9   8   7   6   5   4   3   2   1

Dedication

To our families

Contents

About the Editors

Dr. Joseph Leung is currently the Mr. & Mrs. C.W. Law Professor of Medicine at the University of California, Davis School of Medicine and the Chief of Gastroenterology for the VA Northern California Health Care System. Dr. Leung is a Fellow of the Royal College of Physicians of Edinburgh, Glasgow, and London, as well as the Hong Kong College of Physicians and Hong Kong Academy of Medicine. He is also a Fellow of the American College of Physicians, American College of Gastroenterology, and the American Society for Gastrointestinal Endoscopy.

Dr. Leung has pioneered a number of therapeutic endoscopy procedures including epinephrine injection for ulcer hemostasis, urgent nasobiliary drainage for acute suppurative cholangitis and the design and development of the Cotton-Leung stent for biliary drainage and palliation of malignant obstructive jaundice. Dr. Leung has spent the last 25 years improving ERCP training for GI trainees. He has organized many teaching endoscopy workshops locally, nationally, and internationally and participated as teaching faculty in many more. His current research interests include the use of a mechanical simulator for ERCP training and the impact on clinical performance of beginner trainees.

Dr. Leung received the ACG Senior Governor Award in 2004 and ASGE Master Endoscopist Award in 2005. He was a former Associate Editor for Gastrointestinal Endoscopy and reviewer for a number of prestigious journals including the *New England Journal of Medicine, Gastroenterology, GI Endoscopy,* and the *American Journal of Gastroenterology.* He is the author or coauthor of more than 400 peer-reviewed articles, abstracts, and book chapters, as well as 3 books.

Dr. Simon Lo is Director of the Pancreatic and Biliary Diseases Program at Cedars-Sinai Medical Center, Los Angeles, California.

Contributing Authors

Niraj Ajmere, MD
UMass Memorial Medical Center
Worchester, MA

John Baillie, MB, ChB, FRCP, FACG, FASGE
Wake Forest University Health Sciences
Winston-Salem, NC

Jamie S. Barkin, MD, FACP, MACG, AGAF,
FASGE
Professor of Medicine
University of Miami, Miller School of
Medicine
Chief, Division of Gastroenterology
Mt. Sinai Medical Center
Miami, FL

William R. Brugge, MD
Massachusetts General Hospital
Boston, MA

David L. Carr-Locke, MD, FRCP, FASGE
Brigham & Women's Hospital
Harvard Medical School
Boston, MA

David Cave, MD, PhD
UMass Memorial Medical Center
Worchester, MA

John P. Cello, MD
Professor of Medicine and Surgery
University of California
San Francisco, CA

Kenneth J. Chang, MD, FACG, FASGE
Professor and Chief, Gastroenterology
Director, H. H. Chao Comprehensive Digestive
Disease Center
University of California
Irvine, CA

Christopher J. DiMaio, MD
Assistant Attending Physician
Gastroenterology and Nutrition Service
Memorial Sloan-Kettering Cancer Center
Assistant Professor of Medicine
Weill Medical College of Cornell University
New York, NY

Lynne Do, MD
Clinical Fellow, Division of Gastroenterology
University of California, Davis Medical Center
Sacramento, CA

Francis A. Farraye, MD, MSc
Clinical Director, Section of Gastroenterology
Boston Medical Center
Boston, MA

Erina Foster, MD
Clinical Fellow
Division of Gastroenterology and Hepatology,
University of California, Davis Medical Center
Sacramento, CA

Martin L. Freeman, MD
Professor of Medicine
Director, Pancreaticobiliary Endoscopy
Fellowship Codirector, Minnesota Pancreas
and Liver Center, University of Minnesota
Hennepin County Medical Center
Minneapolis, MN

John S. Goff, MD
Rocky Mountain Gastroenterology Associates
Lakewood, CO

Christopher J. Gostout, MD
Professor of Medicine
Mayo Clinic School of Medicine
Director of Endoscopic Development &
Research
Division of Gastroenterology & Hepatology
Mayo Clinic
Rochester, MN

Rajesh Gupta, MD, DM
Asian Institute of Gastroenterology
Hyderabad, India

Gregory Haber, MD
Director, Division of Gastroenterology,
Center for Advanced Therapeutic Endoscopy,
Lenox Hill Hospital,
New York, NY

Lucinda A. Harris, MS, MD
Assistant Professor of Medicine
College of Medicine, Mayo Clinic
Scottsdale, AZ

Sanjay Hegde, MD
Fox Chase Cancer Center
Gastroenterology Division
Philadelphia, PA

Terry L. Jue, MD
University of California, Davis Medical Center
Sacramento, CA

Michael L. Kochman, MD, FACP
Gastroenterology Division
Hospital of the University of Pennsylvania
Philadelphia, PA

Richard A. Kozarek, MD
Virginia Mason Medical Center
Seattle, WA

John G. Lee, MD
UC Irvine Medical Center
Orange, CA

Jonathan A. Leighton, MD
Professor of Medicine
College of Medicine, Mayo Clinic
Chair, Division of Gastroenterology and
Hepatology
Mayo Clinic
Scottsdale, AZ

Blair S. Lewis, MD
Mt. Sinai Medical Center
Clinical Professor, Gastroenterology
New York, NY

Zhao-shen Li, MD
Changhai Hospital, the Second Military Medical
University
Shanghai, China

Fauze Maluf-Filho, MD, PhD
São Paulo University
São Paulo, SP
Brazil

Nirmal S. Mann, MD, MS, PhD, DSc, FRCPC,
AGAF, FASGE, FACG, MACP
University of California, Davis School of
Medicine
Sacramento, CA

Kanat Ransibrahmanakul, MD
Clinical Fellow, Division of Gastroenterology,
University of California, Davis Medical Center
Sacramento, CA

D. Nageshwar Reddy, MD, DM, FRCP, DSc
Chairman, Asian Institute of Gastroenterology
Hyderabad, India

Paulo Sakai, MD, PhD, FASGE
São Paulo University
São Paulo, SP
Brazil

Thomas J. Savides, MD
Professor of Clinical Medicine
University of California
San Diego, CA

Carol E. Semrad, MD
Associate Professor of Medicine
University of Chicago
Chicago, IL

Stuart Sherman, MD
Professor of Medicine and Radiology
Indiana University Medical Center
Indianapolis, IN

Walter Trudeau, MD
Professor of Medicine
University of California, Davis Medical Center
Sacramento, CA

Jacques Van Dam, MD, PhD
Stanford University Medical Center
Stanford, CA

Hendrikus S. Vanderveldt, MD, MBA
Senior Fellow
University of Miami, Miller School of Medicine
Division of Gastroenterology
Miami, FL

Luo-wei Wang, MD, PhD
Changhai Hospital, the Second Military Medical
University
Shanghai, China

Jerome D. Waye, MD
Mount Sinai Medical Center
New York, NY

Thomas M. Zarchy, MD
USC Keck School of Medicine
Los Angeles, CA

Foreword

We live in the Internet Age—everyone's plugged in, on-line, and busy. Our attention spans have shrunk too, and it's difficult to read textbooks or long journal articles. Still, no matter how pressing our time constraints may be, we must give our patients excellent care even when they pose challenging clinical problems. Thankfully, Drs. Joseph Leung and Simon Lo have written a book that is perfect for endoscopists who are constantly on the go, like me and probably you.

In fact, this excellent tome is best described as a FAQ (frequently asked questions) section for endoscopy. Like the FAQ portion of a Web site, this book saves time by addressing important questions that all gastroenterologists ask from time to time. Unlike most Web sites, though, Drs. Leung and Lo have gathered experts from around the world to answer those questions.

The questions are good ones. From how to handle tough esophageal foreign bodies and pregnant patients to how best to manage recurrent idiopathic pancreatitis and endoscopic perforations, this book provides answers for busy clinicians. The answers are concise and clinically relevant, which helps.

Who are the experts? The table of contents is a few pages back, and a cursory examination of the list of authors will show that Simon and Joseph have assembled a first-rate team. Reading any chapter will reveal that those experts focused on providing answers that are as informative as a reference text and as user-friendly as a curbside consultation from a friend.

Thank you Simon Lo and Joseph Leung for a book that is tailor made for busy endoscopists. It is perfect for the Internet Age.

Stephen M. Schutz, MD
Partner, Boise Digestive Health Clinic
Governor, American College of Gastroenterology
Boise, Idaho

Introduction

Gastroenterology (GI) practice is a diverse and often challenging specialty. Added to the many diagnostic tests is our ability to offer therapeutic endoscopy to treat patients with GI diseases. However, many of these endoscopic procedures are technically challenging, and we often encounter questions related to the application of these techniques in our patients.

Curbside Consultation in Endoscopy: 49 Clinical Questions is set up to provide practicing gastroenterologists with expert opinions and assistance in managing different GI conditions. We have gathered a strong team of therapeutic endoscopists and asked them to share with us their clinical experience in treating patients with tough or recurrent pancreaticobiliary problems and diseases related to the gut. In the different chapters, many experts offer their tricks-of-the-trade with various endoscopy procedures.

For the busy practicing gastroenterologist, this book provides an excellent update on the current management of common GI conditions. For those who are learning to master the skills, they will find that the book offers many practical hints and guidelines for trainees to further improve the care for their patients.

SECTION I

UPPER ENDOSCOPY

AN 81-YEAR-OLD HEALTHY MALE IS FOUND TO HAVE A 12-CM LONG SEGMENT BARRETT'S ESOPHAGUS AND SEVERAL TINY, RAISED LESIONS. BIOPSY SHOWS MODERATE- TO HIGH-GRADE DYSPLASIA IN ONE LOCATION. HOW SHOULD I ADVISE THIS PATIENT ABOUT THIS PROGNOSIS? WHICH SURGICAL OR ENDOSCOPIC THERAPIES WOULD BE APPROPRIATE TO CONSIDER? HOW CAN I TELL WHETHER OR NOT A SMALL CANCER HAS BEEN MISSED IN THE BIOPSY?

Paulo Sakai, MD, PhD, FASGE, and Fauze Maluf-Filho, MD, PhD

Barrett's esophagus (BE) is defined as the presence of specialized columnar metaplasia at the distal esophagus in response to the chronic reflux of gastroduodenal content into the esophagus.

Compared to other patients with gastroesophageal reflux disease, patients with BE present with longer acid and bile exposure. It has been recently acknowledged that the risk of adenocarcinoma associated with BE was overestimated. One case of cancer for approximately 300 patients with BE per year is expected. Long segments of BE (>3 cm) mean a higher risk of cancer when compared to shorter segments. Endoscopic surveillance with routine biopsies is recommended for early detection of adenocarcinoma in these patients. The presence of cellular atypia confined to the epithelium is called dysplasia and is considered to be a marker for the development of invasive adenocarcinoma in BE. When high-grade dysplasia (HGD) is detected and confirmed by a senior pathologist, the patient should be made aware of the 30% to 40% risk that an invasive adenocarcinoma was missed in the endoscopy. The incidence of cancer after diagnosis of HGD may be in approximately 28% to 30% of the patients, which definitely is an indication for treatment.[1] Controversy exists regarding the optimal management of BE with HGD. There are two options: 1) esophagectomy to prevent cancer and cure early cancer and 2) endoscopic ablation and resection to remove the neoplastic mucosa to prevent cancer and cure mucosal cancer.

For some investigators, particularly among surgeons, BE with HGD has been considered an indication for esophagectomy because of the increased risk of cancer. The patient should be referred to high-volume surgical consultation centers where more than 50 esophagectomies are performed every year. In these centers, the mortality rate related to this extensive surgery is lower than 5%. However, the endoscopic therapy may be an attractive and less invasive treatment alternative since the risk of lymph node involvement or hematogenous dissemination is absent in HGD and negligible in early stage cancer. Endoscopic therapy may be performed through local endoscopic mucosal resection or through endoscopic ablation using photodynamic therapy (PDT), argon plasma coagulation (APC), or radiofrequency ablation (RFA).

Endoscopic mucosal resection (EMR) is safe and effective for complete HGD local resection and early BE cancer. Usually two endoscopic techniques are applied: cap-technique and band-ligation technique (Figure 1-1). In both techniques, piecemeal resection is required when the lesion is larger than 10 to 15 mm. More recently, another technique called endoscopic submucosal dissection (ESD) is being used for the resection of a large lesion *en bloc*, but specific accessories and training are required for this procedure. For BE more than 3 cm in length, the complete circumferential removal of the mucosa may cause an esophageal stricture. One of the most frequently studied endoscopic therapies for HGD in BE is photodynamic therapy. It is an expensive method of limited availability, and long-term results are not well described. There is a 40% rate of esophageal stenosis, and small foci of invasive cancer may be left untreated. Ablative therapy such as PDT and APC do not provide a specimen for histopathological evaluation, and usually the depth of eradication is limited. Residual BEs under restored squamous epithelium after endoscopic tissue ablative therapy may occur in 20% to 30% of cases. The use of RFA seems to be very effective, but long-term evaluation is not yet available.[2]

With a 12-cm long segment BE and several raised lesions with HGD in a healthy person, the esophagectomy could be considered. Although preoperative morbidity is significant, surgical resection of HGD in BE may provide excellent long-term survival with acceptable quality of life.[3] On the other hand, the endoscopic resection may be another option. All lesions may be locally resected although in the remaining BE, approximately 11% of patients will have a recurrence or development of metachronous HGD or an early stage cancer in a long-term follow-up, and these can be treated again through endoscopic

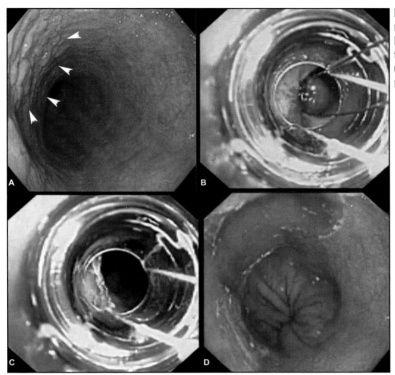

Figure 1-1. (A) Long segment of BE with HGD lesion, (B, C) band-ligation mucosectomy and (D) final aspect of local resection.

resection.[4] Therefore, we emphasize the importance of a strict endoscopic follow-up in order to detect and treat any recurrent lesion. Ideally, all possible columnar mucosa with intestinal metaplasia should be eradicated and this approach would be recommended in patients with invisible or multiple neoplastic areas in a shorter BE.

In conclusion, we can offer for this patient two options: 1) esophagectomy as a definite treatment and 2) endoscopic resection of HGD lesions with less morbidity but with the need for a strict endoscopic follow-up.

Reference

1. Wang KK, Wongkeesong M, Buttar NS. American Gastroenterological Association medical position statement: Role of the gastroenterologist in the management of esophageal carcinoma. *Gastroenterology.* 2005;128:1468-1470.
2. Sharma VK, Wang KK, Overholt BF, et al. Balloon-based, circumferential, endoscopic radiofrequency ablation of Barrett´s esophagus: 1-year follow-up of 100 patients. *Gastrointest Endosc.* 2007;65:185-195.
3. Headrick JR, Nichols III FC, Miller DL, et al. High-grade esophageal dysplasia: long-term survival and quality of life after esophagectomy. *Ann Thorac Surg.* 2002;73:1697-1703.
4. Ell C, May A, Pech O, et al. Curative endoscopic resection of early esophageal adenocarcinomas (Barrett´s cancer). *Gastrointest Endosc.* 2007;65:3-10.

Is Endoscopic Biopsy of the Duodenum or Jejunum Necessary for the Diagnosis of Celiac Disease if the Serum Anti-Tissue Transglutaminase Antibody Is Positive? Is Capsule Endoscopy Good Enough to Make the Diagnosis? When and How Should I Investigate for Complications of Celiac Disease?

Carol E. Semrad, MD

Celiac disease is an inflammatory disease of the small bowel that is triggered by gluten (wheat, rye, barley) in the diet in a genetically susceptible host (HLA-DQ2, -DQ8, and other genes). Some patients present with diarrhea and weight loss or atypical signs; others are asymptomatic and detected incidentally at endoscopy or by antibody screening. Small bowel biopsy is not specific for celiac disease. Biopsy findings range from mild inflammation, Marsh I classification (increased intraepithelial lymphocytes), to severe inflammation, Marsh III classification (increased intraepithelial and lamina propria lymphocytes, increased plasma cells, villous atrophy, and crypt hyperplasia). The diagnosis of celiac disease is made when there is clinical or biopsy improvement while on a gluten-free diet.

Over the years, a number of antibodies have been identified that are associated with celiac disease with varying sensitivities and specificities. Anti-gliadin antibodies are the least specific and should no longer be used in the diagnosis of adult disease. Endomysial antibody (EMA) nears 100% specificity but its sensitivity can vary (an indirect immuno-fluorescence study that requires technical expertise). The antigen recognized by the endo-mysial antibody, tissue transglutaminase (tTG), has been identified. This has resulted in the development of the tTG immunoglobulin A (IgA) enzyme-linked immunosorbent assay (ELISA) antibody assay that is highly sensitive but less specific than EMA. The tTG IgA test is not interpretable in IgA deficient individuals with very low IgA levels. False positive tTG antibody studies have been reported in Crohn's disease, primary biliary cirrhosis, and other autoimmune diseases.

Although a positive tTG and EMA antibody study together is highly specific for celiac disease, a duodenal biopsy is still recommended for diagnosis. The treatment of celiac disease is a life-long gluten-free diet. Adherence is difficult because wheat is ubiquitous in foods, particularly processed and restaurant foods. Some fail to improve on a gluten-free diet, raising the question of a correct diagnosis. In addition, when the reality of a life-long gluten-free diet sets in, those with milder symptoms may question their diagnosis. The more secure the diagnosis (positive tTG/EMA antibodies, abnormal small bowel biopsy, HLA-DQ2 or -DQ8 genotype), the easier it is to reinforce the need for a gluten-free diet until other therapies are available. A secure diagnosis also sets into motion antibody screening of other family members for celiac disease.

In those who cannot undergo small bowel biopsy, the diagnosis of celiac disease should never be made by a positive tTG antibody study alone without confirmation of a positive EMA test. A false positive tTG antibody test may result in the wrong diagnosis.

Is Capsule Endoscopy Good Enough to Make the Diagnosis?

Video capsule endoscopy is a new technology that allows visualization of the entire small bowel but lacks capability for small bowel biopsy. It has been reported to have good sensitivity and high specificity in the detection of severe villous atrophy in celiac disease. Characteristic findings include decreased duodenal/jejunal folds and mucosal scalloping, fissuring, or mosaic pattern. However, not all villous atrophy is due to celiac disease, and some individuals with celiac disease have mild inflammation without atrophy, hence normal appearing small bowel mucosa. Therefore, some cases of celiac disease will be missed. Video capsule endoscopy is a diagnostic alternative in those who have a positive EMA antibody and refuse or cannot undergo small bowel biopsy. Follow-up studies for improvement in mucosal appearance on a gluten-free diet have not been performed.

When and How Should I Investigate for Complications of Celiac Disease?

The first consideration is to assess for possible vitamin and mineral deficiencies. Celiac disease usually affects the proximal small intestine, the site of highest exposure to ingested gluten. Nutrients most likely to be malabsorbed include iron, folate, and calcium because their carrier proteins have highest or exclusive expression in the proximal small bowel. A bone mineral density study should be obtained. About 60% of those with celiac disease have bone mass loss; men often have greater loss than women. Anemia due to malaborption of iron is common. An improvement in anemia and bone density is a good indication of recovery on a gluten-free diet. There is no role for bisphosphonates early in the treatment of celiac disease. Bone mass often improves on a gluten-free diet alone, and hypocalcemia may occur in those with severe disease and poor calcium absorption.

Those with severe diarrhea or weight loss may have inflammation of the entire small intestine. Such individuals are at risk for fluid and electrolyte, fat soluble and B12 vitamin, and zinc deficiencies. Vitamin B12 and zinc are necessary for regeneration of the intestinal epithelium. Failure to replete these nutrients may delay mucosal recovery on a gluten-free diet in severe cases.

Individuals with celiac disease who fail to improve on a gluten-free diet need further investigation. First, strictness of a gluten-free diet needs to be scrutinized by a knowledgeable dietician. If the diet is strict, persistent diarrhea may be due to a missed diagnosis, bacterial overgrowth, pancreatic insufficiency (failure to release secretin/CCK from an atrophied small bowel mucosa), or microscopic colitis. The small bowel biopsy should be reviewed by an expert pathologist for a possible missed diagnosis, commonly infection and agammaglobulinemia. Autoimmune enteropathy is very rare and occur mainly in children. It is characterized by a positive anti-enterocyte and anti-goblet cell antibodies with loss of goblet cells and increased crypt apoptosis on small bowel biopsy.

When there is no response to a gluten-free diet for over 12 months or alarm symptoms (abdominal pain, diarrhea weight loss) occur after previous response to a gluten-free diet, refractory celiac disease should be considered. Diagnosis requires special histochemical studies on formalin fixed small bowel biopsy tissue including T-cell markers and T-cell receptor gamma gene rearrangements. Refractory celiac disease type I is characterized by a normal population of T cells (CD3+, CD8+), a good response to immunosuppressive agents, and a good prognosis. Type II is characterized by an abnormal population of T cells (CD3+, CD8-), a poor response to immunosuppressive agents, frequent progression to T-cell lymphoma, and a poor prognosis. Video capsule endoscopy may be useful to screen for T-cell lymphoma or ulcerative jejunitis. In those with suspicious lesions deep in the small bowel, double balloon enteroscopy is of value in obtaining a tissue diagnosis.

References

1. Green PHR, Cellier C. Celiac disease. *NEJM*. 2007;357:1731-1743.
2. Al-toma A, Verbeek WHM, Mulder CJJ. Update on the management of refractory celiac disease. *J Gastrointestin Liver Dis*. 2007;16:57-63.
3. Rondonotti E, Spada C, Cave D, et al. Video capsule enteroscopy in the diagnosis of celiac disease: a multi-center study. *Am J Gastroenterol*. 2007;102:1624-1631.
4. Hadithi M, Al-toma A, Oudejans J, et al. The value of double-balloon enteroscopy in patients with refractory celiac disease. *Am J Gastroenterol*. 2007;102:987-996.

A 46-Year-Old Female With Cirrhosis Came in With Severe Upper GI Bleeding. Her Proximal Stomach Is Filled With Large Clots and Gastric Varices Are Suspected. How Can I Tell for Certain Endoscopically, and How Should I Treat It?

Kanat Ransibrahmanakul, MD, and
Joseph Leung, MD, FRCP, FACP, FACG, FASGE

This patient presumably presents with severe upper gastrointestinal bleeding (UGIB). To help determine the cause of bleeding, one should conduct an initial clinical assessment including a history and physical exam. The history may reveal common causes of bleeding such as peptic ulcer disease, Mallory-Weiss tear, esophagitis,[1] and esophageal/gastric varices. Particular attention is paid to look for stigmata of chronic liver disease such as spider angiomata, ascites, and palmar erythema. Laboratory studies may reveal thrombocytopenia and elevated international normalized ratio (INR) as a result of cirrhosis and chronic liver disease. If bleeding from varices is suspected, intravenous octreotide 50 μg bolus should be given followed by octreotide drip 50 μg per hour and continued until endoscopy is performed. If endoscopy confirms variceal hemorrhage, the octreotide drip should be continued for at least another 72 hours. Early use of proton pump inhibitors (PPIs) should also be considered if the cause of bleeding is unclear. Appropriate

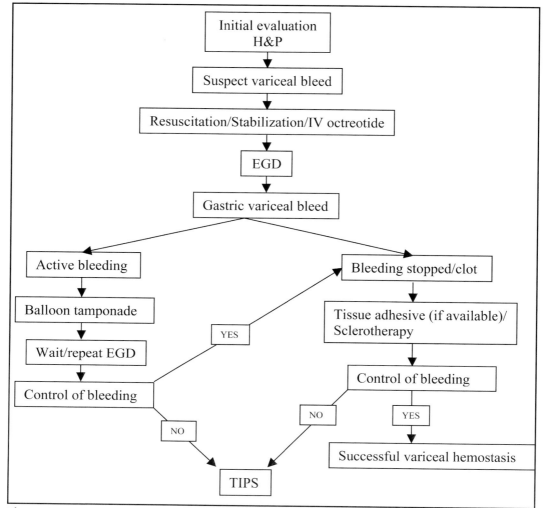

Figure 3-1. Approach to a patient with possible gastric variceal bleeding.

antibiotics such as intravenous ciprofloxacin or ceftriaxone should be given in all cirrhotic patients with gastrointestinal (GI) hemorrhage for short-term prophylaxis against spontaneous bacterial peritonitis.

Before attempting esophagogastroduodenoscopy (EGD), the patient must be appropriately resuscitated and stabilized. Orthostatic changes in blood pressure and pulse implies at least a 15% reduction in circulating blood volume. With all GI bleeds, two large bore intravenous (IV) tubes must be placed and fluids and blood products given to stabilize the patient hemodynamically. Correcting any underlying bleeding tendency will help with hemostasis. Significant upper GI bleeding warrants airway protection including elective intubation prior to emergency endoscopy. Furthermore, the patient should be admitted to the intensive care unit (ICU) for monitoring.

If urgent endoscopy reveals presence of large clots in the proximal stomach and evidence of active bleeding that impair visualization, and if gastric varices are suspected, balloon tamponade should be used in an attempt to achieve initial hemostasis. Either a Sengstaken-Blakemore tube or Minnesota tube should be placed with the gastric balloon inflated inside the stomach and pulled with adequate pressure against the gastric fundus to achieve tamponade. After waiting a few hours, repeat endoscopy should then be performed.

Suctioning is ineffective in removing clots as these can block the relatively small suction channel of the endoscope. Clots can be removed using a large bore gastric lavage tube with copious irrigation and siphonage. If upper endoscopy reveals that the bleeding has stopped and the views are satisfactory, endoscopic procedures may be performed. To assist in cleansing the stomach for optimal endoscopy, intravenous erythromycin 250 mg or metoclopramide 10 mg can be given 30 minutes prior to the endoscopy. Attempts can be made to remove any overlying clots by additional endoscopic irrigation. Repositioning of the patient to the right lateral position may help to move the clots away from the fundus for better visualization. Once the clots are removed, appropriate endoscopic therapy can be performed. In stable patients where the diagnosis of gastric varices is in doubt, endoscopic ultrasound is helpful to clarify the diagnosis.

If gastric varices are deemed to be the source of bleeding, gastric variceal obliteration with tissue adhesives should be attempted where available. N-butyl-2-cyanoacrylate is available for use in Europe and Asia. In the United States, 2-octyl cyanoacrylate has been approved by the FDA for tissue closure and has been reported to be effective for achieving initial hemostasis and preventing rebleeding from fundal varices.[1] The technique requires technical skill and caution to avoid damage to the endoscope. However, complications, although rare, may include embolic events (ie, cerebral stroke, portal vein embolism, splenic infarction, cardiac emboli and pulmonary embolism associated with the cyanoacrylate injections).[2] To prevent glue sticking and damage to the endoscope, lipiodol should be used to coat the tip of the endoscope and flush the biopsy channel. A disposable sclerotherapy injection needle and catheter should be primed and preloaded with a mixture of 1:1 cyanoacrylate and lipiodol prior to insertion into the endoscope.[3] After puncturing the varix lumen with the needle, the tissue adhesive is injected in 1 mL aliquots by using normal saline solution to flush the tissue adhesive into the varix until the varix is firm to palpation with the tip of the catheter.[2]

Gastric varices are classified as gastroesophageal varices and isolated gastric varices. Gastric varices coexisting with esophageal varices are type 1 gastroesophageal varices (GOV1), which extend along the lesser curvature, and type 2 gastroesophageal varices (GOV2), which extend to the greater curvature. Isolated gastric varices are type 1 isolated gastric varices (IGV1), existing only in the fundus, and type 2 isolated gastric varices (IGV2), existing sporadically.[4] Sclerotherapy has been more successful in GOV than IGV.[5] Injection of sclerosants may be performed using the intravariceal or paravariceal injection technique. Important complications of endoscopic sclerotherapy include fever, retrosternal pain, dysphagia, injection-induced bleeding, ulceration, perforation, mediastinitis, pleural effusion, fistula, adult respiratory distress syndrome, and infectious complications.[6]

Transjugular intrahepatic portosystemic shunt (TIPS) has been shown to be highly effective for control of gastric variceal hemorrhage. Threshold for TIPS placement for bleeding from gastric varices should be lower than bleeding from esophageal varices and TIPS should be placed if endoscopic therapy is not possible or after a failed attempt of endoscopic treatment.[7]

In summary, management of this cirrhotic patient who presents with severe upper GI bleeding from suspected gastric varices should include appropriate initial evaluation, resuscitation, and stabilization. The patient should be admitted to the ICU for close monitoring, including potential tracheal intubation for airway protection prior to endoscopy. Judicious transfusions of blood products and appropriate antibiotics should be given. Balloon tamponade should be considered if the patient is actively bleeding in order to achieve initial hemostasis. IV erythromycin should be given prior to the endoscopy to improve visualization during endoscopy. The gastric varices should be classified into either gastroesophageal varices or isolated gastric varices, which may be useful in predicting the response to endoscopic therapy.

Fundal gastric varices should be treated with pharmacological and endoscopic therapy, and tissue adhesives should be used if available. TIPS should be considered if endoscopic therapy is not amendable or if bleeding recurs.

References

1. Rengstorff DS, Binmoeller KF. A pilot study of 2-octyl cyanoacrylate injection for treatment of gastric fundal varices in humans. *Gastrointest Endosc.* 2004;59:553-558.
2. Tripathi D, Ferguson JW, Therapondos G, et al. Review article: recent advances in the management of bleeding gastric varices. *Aliment Pharmacol Ther.* 2006;24:1-17.
3. Dhiman RK, Chawla Y, Taneja S, et al. Endoscopic sclerotherapy of gastric variceal bleeding with N-butyl-2-cyanoacrylate. *J Clin Gastroenterol.* 2002;35:222-227.
4. Sarin SK, Lahoti D, Saxena SP, Murthy NS, Makwana UK. Prevalence, classification and natural history of gastric varices: a long-term follow-up study in 568 portal hypertension patients. *Hepatology.* 1992;16:1343-1349.
5. Park WG, Yeh RW, Triadafilopoulos G. Injection therapies for variceal bleeding disorders of the GI tract. *Gastrointest Endosc.* 2008;67:313-323.
6. Qureshi W, Adler DG, Davila R, et al. ASGE Guideline: the role of endoscopy in the management of variceal hemorrhage, updated July 2005. *Gastrointest Endosc.* 2005;62:651-655.
7. Garcia-Tsao G, Sanyal AJ, Grace ND, Carey WD. Prevention and management of gastroesophageal varices and variceal hemorrhage in cirrhosis. *Am J Gastroenterol.* 2007;102:2086-2102.

IS MY IMPRESSION CORRECT THAT ENDOSCOPIC GERD TREATMENT IS A THING OF THE PAST? IF SO, WHY? FOR WHICH ENDOSCOPIC METHOD SHOULD I REFER PATIENTS?

Christopher J. Gostout, MD

Endoscopic treatment is not a thing of the past. The concept is alive and progress is actually continuing in this area. Endolumenal therapies for GERD have suffered for a variety of reasons. These include: marginal long-term control of symptoms and elimination of PPI use, lack of support by the academic community, and perhaps most importantly, the lack of a billing code acceptable to Medicare and insurers. There remain only two commercially available endolumenal therapies—the Endocinch device (C. R. Bard, Inc., Murray Hill, NJ) and the NDO full-thickness plicator (NDO Surgical, Inc., Mansfield, MA). There are several newer technologies undergoing development, with one nearing approval by the United States Food and Drug Administration (FDA).

The Endocinch device was the very first endolumenal therapy to surface. The currently available device remains cumbersome to use, requiring two endoscopes and multiple intubations. The durability of the suture plication is highly variable. These issues limit the value of the procedure and effectively have eliminated popular use. The device is undergoing modification that will allow single intubation without need for an overtube, and allow multiple stitches, even full thickness in depth. Once this modified device is available, it may result in a renewed interest.

The NDO full thickness plicator can provide effective treatment for uncomplicated GERD for up to 5 years. There is an ongoing effort to summarize 5-year outcomes in the group of patients treated during the original pivotal trial. Some have advocated the placement of more than one plication for more effective symptom control; however, this has not prevailed. The device is large and very difficult to pass comfortably through the pharynx and upper esophageal sphincter in any patient. Therefore, the procedure is best performed with the assistance of anesthesia, if not formal endotracheal intubation. The current device allows only one plication to be created per intubation. Outcomes are operator dependent and specifically are dependent on careful placement of the suture-based implant close to the squamocolumnar junction. The procedure is safe. With the need for anesthesia, the procedure becomes expensive. The major limitation of this therapy is the lack of reimbursement by insurers.

The endolumenal fundoplication (ELF) procedure using the EsophyX device (Endogastric Solutions, WA) holds promise to become the endoscopic procedure of choice. The procedure is designed to create an internal sphincter within the cardia that recreates a robust angle of HIS (the gastroesophageal junctional angle between the cardia and fundus). The valve (average 4 cm in length) is built by invaginating the gastric wall, full thickness (serosa to serosa), nearly circumferentially around the cardia, sparing only the lesser curve. This is accomplished by placing multiple (8 to 12) "H"-shaped tissue anchors through the inverted gastric wall drawn into the device. The device is also designed to allow reduction of small hiatal hernias (≤ 2 cm). Similar to the other types of plication-type methods, the procedure is performed with the endoscope in a retroflexed position, using a standard diagnostic endoscope. This procedure is designed to be performed under general anesthesia in an operating room. Since this has been developed as a surgical procedure, attempting to mimic the Hill repair, it will be subject to surgical billing and ultimately should be much more successful from the standpoint of reimbursement. The device and procedure have been tested in over 250 patients. The device is commercially available and in use in Europe. This is the only endoscopic anti-reflux procedure that has been able to effectively demonstrate normalization of pH, in addition to consistent elimination of PPI use. Patient follow-up is approaching 2 years with this new method.

In summary, there remains a role for endoscopic endolumenal GERD therapies. These therapies can be strongly considered in the following situations: as an adjunctive therapy to PPIs, for control of regurgitation in patients who have their pyrosis effectively controlled with PPIs, and select patient groups. One patient group involves the scleroderma patient who is not a candidate for a Nissen fundoplication. Patients with non-acid reflux are also another group of potential candidates for endoscopic therapy. Patients troubled with regurgitation and controlled pyrosis on PPIs comprise the largest group of patients in my practice.

Reference

1. Cadiere GB, Rajan A, Rqibate M, et al. Endoluminal fundoplication (ELF)- evolution of EsophyX, a new surgical device for transoral surgery. *Minimally Invasive Therapy*. 2006;15(6):348-355.

WHAT ARE THE RECOMMENDATIONS FOR PERFORMING ENDOSCOPY—AND ESPECIALLY ERCP—IN A PREGNANT WOMAN?

John Baillie, MB, ChB, FRCP, FACG, FASGE

When a pregnant woman is referred for an endoscopic procedure, the first question one should ask is "how necessary is this test?" Beyond the first trimester, most pregnancies are as solid as the Rock of Gibraltar, but we still need to avoid unnecessary sedation, instrumentation, and irradiation of pregnant women. Clearly, medical emergencies such as an acute abdominal pain, ingested foreign body, hematemesis, and hematochezia demand urgent evaluation. Less clamant problems, such as chronic abdominal pain, can almost always be investigated without endoscopy and managed symptomatically. No pregnant woman needs sphincter of Oddi (SO) manometry in a search for biliary dyskinesia or colonoscopy to investigate constipation. Heartburn and epigastric pain that respond to antacids can be managed this way and do not require esophagogastroduo-denoscopy (EGD). Flexible sigmoidoscopy, typically performed without sedation, is an appropriate and benign investigation during pregnancy for nonresolving diarrhea and minor rectal bleeding. Rarely, therapeutic endoscopy may be required to treat an actively bleeding ulcer or esophageal varices during pregnancy. In such circumstances, the mother's life is at risk and concerns for the health of the fetus must be secondary. Although EGD and colonoscopy are generally considered safe in pregnancy, this opinion is based on scant data with very few published series. The decision to employ endoscopy during pregnancy should be made on a case-by-case basis with a solid justification for each procedure. Some guidelines cite pregnancy as a contraindication to performing capsule endoscopy, and there are no data on the safety of double balloon enteroscopy in this setting. The most invasive endoscopic procedure performed during pregnancy is endoscopic retrograde cholangiopancreatography (ERCP).

Indications for ERCP in Pregnancy

The most frequent indications for ERCP in pregnancy are the management of common bile duct stones (choledocholithiasis) causing biliary colic, obstructive jaundice or pancreatitis, and the identification and treatment of bile duct leaks post-cholecystectomy. Surgeons wish to avoid cholecystectomy in the first trimester of pregnancy, as it is associated with risk of fetal loss. The first trimester uterus is easily shielded against radiation, and patient positioning is rarely a problem. If it appears that the "offending" bile duct stone has already passed, as evidenced by the rapid rise and fall of liver enzymes (eg, alanine aminotransferase) over the first 24 to 48 hours, it is safer to perform intraoperative cholangiography (IOC) at the time of surgery than to subject the patient to the risks of ERCP (mainly acute pancreatitis). Only a positive IOC requires follow-up ERCP. Known bile duct stones identified by ultrasound, IOC, endoscopic ultrasound (EUS), or magnetic resonance cholangiopancreatography (MRCP) should not be left to pass spontaneously, as there is always a risk (albeit small) of acute gallstone pancreatitis when this happens. Pancreatitis in pregnancy in patients who do not appear to have gallstones on standard imaging techniques may be due to biliary microlithiasis. EUS is the most sensitive way to detect this, and the "cure" is cholecystectomy. ERCP is generally not recommended during pregnancy to define the pancreatic ductal anatomy. Endoscopic decompression of a pancreatic pseudocyst (aspiration ± drainage) would be preferable to placing a percutaneous drain or performing surgery during pregnancy. However, the author is not aware of any reported case of this use of ERCP or EUS. Bile duct leaks following cholecystectomy during pregnancy are managed in the standard fashion, by endoscopic stenting or biliary sphincterotomy. In this situation, intra-abdominal fluid collections large enough to drain percutaneously should be sought by transcutaneous ultrasound examination or cross-sectional imaging (eg, MRI). Bilomas can become infected or extend into the peritoneal cavity, causing peritonitis; it should never be assumed that a bilioma will resolve spontaneously.

Informed Consent

Informed consent for ERCP in pregnancy should cover the commonly recognized complications (ie, perforation, bleeding, pancreatitis, infection) as well as the potential for fetal distress or loss. The precautions being taken to minimize exposure to ionizing radiation (see below) should be explained to the patient. If general anesthesia (with or without endotracheal intubation) is going to be used for the procedure, the anesthesia provider should obtain separate informed consent for this.

Positioning for ERCP

Positioning for ERCP is typically prone or semiprone in the first trimester. In the second and (especially) third trimesters, pregnant women are most comfortable lying on their side. The supine position should be avoided in late pregnancy to avoid compression of the aorta and (especially) inferior vena cava by the gravid uterus, which may cause supine hypotension syndrome (due to interference with venous return from the lower limbs). The requirements of the anesthesiologist often differ from those of the endoscopist, so the two should confer and agree on positioning ahead of time. It is essential to

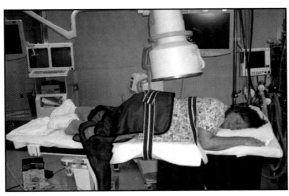

Figure 5-1. Pregnant woman positioned on fluoroscopy table in preparation for ERCP. A lead apron is being used to shield the fetus.

know which direction x-rays will travel (ie, from above to below the x-ray table, or vice versa) so that lead shielding (typically a lead apron) can be positioned appropriately to shield the fetus (Figure 5-1). A radiation dosimeter should be placed under the shielding and over the gravid uterus to measure actual radiation exposure during the procedure.

To Intubate or Not Intubate?

Gastroesophageal reflux of gastric contents is common during pregnancy, related to hormonal changes that slow gastric emptying and relax the esophageal sphincters. The tendency to reflux is also related to intra-abdominal pressure from the gravid uterus. Anesthesiologists consider pregnant women to be at risk for aspiration events, especially in the later stages of pregnancy. As pulmonary aspiration of gastric contents can be a catastrophic event, most anesthesiologists want to protect the airway by endotracheal intubation. This is a wise precaution in pregnant women undergoing potentially long procedures, such as ERCP and EUS. The timing and manner of removing the endotracheal tube requires care in these patients, an issue of which anesthesiologists and their support personnel are well aware. Unsedated endoscopy (including transnasal endoscopy) is feasible for EGD in some pregnant women but is unrealistic for ERCP, which is rarely "quick."

Fetal Monitoring

Fetal monitoring is appropriate immediately before and after the procedure to ensure the health of the fetus, but is not required during ERCP.

Fluoroscopy for ERCP

Fluoroscopy for ERCP should be kept to an absolute minimum. Short (ie, seconds at a time) bursts of fluoroscopy are all that are required to confirm the position of the cannula within the desired duct (usually the common bile duct) and to identify pathology after injection of contrast medium. Digital fluoroscopy allows capture of fluoroscopic images to provide a "hard copy" record of the procedure with low levels of radiation exposure. A radiation dosimeter is typically placed on the patient's abdomen just above the protective lead shield and another one beneath the shield over the expected position of the fetus.

The radiation exposure is typically minimal, but the results should be kept as part of the patient's record.

COMPLICATIONS OF ERCP

Complications of ERCP during pregnancy are (thankfully) rare, which likely reflects the skill of the endoscopists to whom pregnant women are referred and care with which they choose their cases. The most feared complication of ERCP is severe (necrotizing) acute pancreatitis, which could threaten the life of both mother and unborn child. Temporary stenting of the pancreatic duct to minimize the risk of necrotizing pancreatitis should be considered whenever there has been extensive manipulation of the duodenal papilla and/or repeated instrumentation of the pancreatic duct. A pancreatic stent designed to dislodge spontaneously (eg, a single pigtail, 3-5 French gauge stent with a single—or no—internal flap) will avoid the need for repeat endoscopy.

References

1. Cappell MS. Safety of endoscopy in pregnancy. *Nature Clin Pract Gastroenterol Hepatol.* 2005;2:376-377.
2. Qureshi WA, Rajan E, Adler DG, et al. ASGE guideline: guidelines for endoscopy in pregnant and lactating women. *Gastrointest Endosc.* 2005;61(3):357-362.
3. Tham TC, Vandervoort JC, Wong RC, et al. Safety of ERCP in pregnancy. *Am J Gastroenterol.* 2003;98(2):308-311.

WHAT ARE THE ESSENTIAL TOOLS FOR REMOVING ESOPHAGOGASTRIC FOREIGN BODIES, AND WHEN SHOULD I APPLY THESE DEVICES?

Luo-wei Wang, MD, PhD, and Zhao-shen Li, MD

Foreign-object ingestion and food-bolus impaction occur commonly. The majority of foreign bodies (ie, foreign objects and food-bolus) that reach the stomach will pass spontaneously. However, 10% to 20% of cases will require nonoperative intervention and approximately 1% will require surgical procedures.[1] Most cases of foreign body ingestion occur in the pediatric age group, with a peak incidence between 6 months and 6 years.[2] In adults, foreign object ingestion occurs more commonly among patients with psychiatric illnesses, mental retardation, alcoholic intoxication, pica, and those seeking secondary gain with access to a medical facility.[3,4]

Since the first report in 1972 on the removal of a foreign body with a flexible endoscope by McKechnie,[5] there has been an increasing application of this method because of its advantages: avoidance of operations/surgeries for most patients, a reduced cost, easy accessibility to the esophagus with endoscopy, excellent visualization and simultaneous diagnosis of underlying diseases, a low morbidity, etc.

Preparation Before Endoscopic Removal of Foreign Bodies

Prior to endoscopic extraction of a foreign body, information regarding the type, form, and size of the foreign body is required to plan the strategy of removal and to select the appropriate instruments. If necessary, it may be useful to conduct a dry run of the

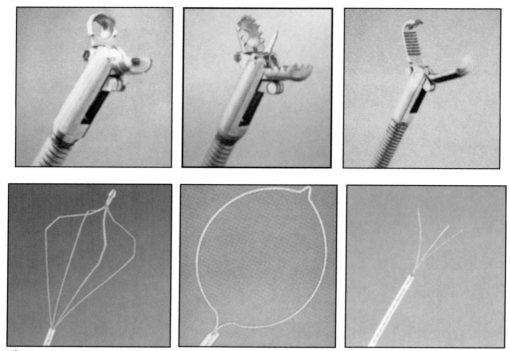

Figure 6-1. Accessories used to remove foreign bodies.

procedure before performing it on the patient. A plain radiograph of the upper GI tract with contrast study may be necessary. If a perforation is suspected, water-soluble contrast such as Gastrografin (Bracco Diagnostics, Inc., Princeton, NJ) is preferred. If an esophageal foreign body is suspected, a plain x-ray of the chest including the neck region should be taken to rule out foreign bodies impacted at the cricopharyngeal sphincter. Children and uncooperative adults often require endotracheal intubation and general anesthesia to insure that the procedure is carried out safely and successfully.

Endoscopes and Accessories

Standard flexible endoscopes are used in adult patients. A smaller, flexible nasoendoscope with an outer diameter of 6 mm and a special oral retainer is used in children less than 3 years. A double-channel endoscope is used to extract complex and ultra long objects such as dental prostheses and chopsticks. Accessories used to remove foreign bodies included rat-tooth forceps, snare, W-shaped forceps, retrieval basket, tripod forceps, biopsy forceps, and alligator jaws forceps (Figure 6-1). A latex protector hood (Figure 6-2) or an overtube (Figure 6-3) is used to protect the upper GI tract during removal of sharp foreign bodies. Patients with psychiatric illness need general anesthesia with close monitoring of the heart rate and blood pressure. Other patients may need IV sedation with diazepam when necessary.

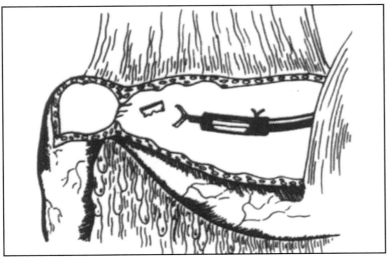

Figure 6-2. Latex protector hood during removal of sharp foreign bodies.

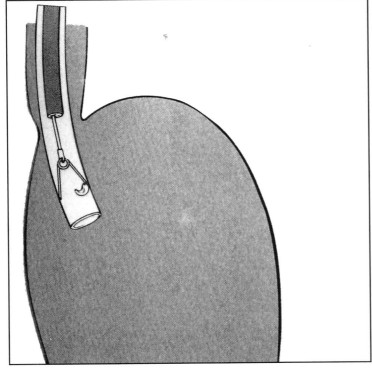

Figure 6-3. Remove sharp foreign bodies with the overtube.

WHEN SHOULD I APPLY ENDOSCOPY AND THESE ACCESSORIES?

Standard and therapeutic endoscopes are used. Equipment that is essential includes rat-tooth and alligator forceps, polypectomy snare, polyp grasper, retrieval net, overtubes of esophageal and gastric lengths, and a foreign body protector hood. Different endoscopic methods and equipment are used depending on the types of foreign bodies. Food bolus can usually be removed en bloc (Figure 6-4) or in a piecemeal fashion

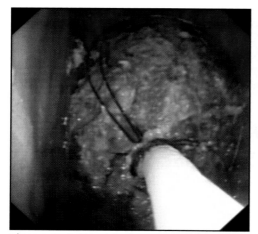

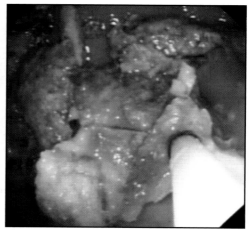

Figure 6-4. Food bolus removed en bloc using the retrieval basket.

Figure 6-5. Food bolus removed in a piece-meal fashion using the retrieval basket.

Figure 6-6. Coins removed with rat-tooth forceps.

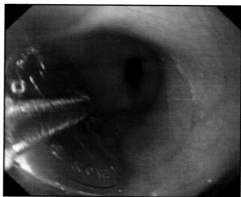

using the retrieval basket (Figure 6-5), rat-tooth forceps, or snare. When the endoscope, upon air insufflation and distention of the esophageal lumen, can be steered around the food bolus and into the stomach, the endoscope can be pulled back and used to gently push the food bolus into the stomach. Food boluses should always be pushed carefully into the stomach under direct vision. Coins can be removed easily with a foreign body forceps (Figure 6-6) (rat-tooth, alligator jaws), a snare, or retrieval net.[6] Fish bones (Figure 6-7) and dental prostheses (Figure 6-8) are sharp pointed objects commonly ingested by adults and elderly men. Sharp-pointed objects lodged in the esophagus present a medical emergency. Endoscopic retrieval of these sharp objects is accomplished with retrieval forceps (rat-tooth or alligator jaws forceps) or a snare. The risk of mucosal injury during sharp-object retrieval can be minimized by orienting the object with the point trailing during extraction and by using an overtube or a protector hood attached to the end of the endoscope. Webb reported a 98.8% success rate of endoscopic removal of foreign bodies and a 1.2% failure rate.[6] Li et al reported a success rate for removal of esophageal foreign bodies with a flexible endoscope in 94.1% of cases with a failure rate of 5.9%.[7] Most of the foreign bodies that fail endoscopic removal are dental prostheses, iron slices, or complex

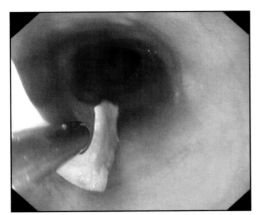 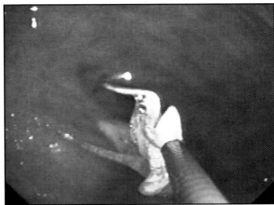

Figure 6-7. Fish bones removed with rat-tooth forceps.

Figure 6-8. Dental prostheses removed with snare.

and ultra-long objects. Dental prostheses always impact into the esophageal mucosa, usually involving the muscular layer. In clinical practice, if the risk of esophageal perforation and bleeding is high, as in those cases with dental prostheses deeply embedded into the esophageal wall, it is better to avoid endoscopic attempts and to refer the patient directly to surgery.

Long foreign objects are difficult to remove endoscopically because of difficulty in orientation and grasping. In a retrospective analysis of 542 cases of foreign body ingestion, Velitchkov et al found that all 17 spoon handles longer than 6 cm remained within the stomach and required surgical removal.[8]

Complications

A complication rate of up to 5% is reported for endoscopic treatment including mucosal laceration, bleeding, pyrexia, and in severe cases, esophageal perforation.[9] The mucosal laceration and bleeding can be treated immediately by endoscopy. Patients with pyrexia should be covered with antibiotics for 2 days. However, patients with esophageal perforation will need surgery.

References

1. Eisen GM, Baron TH, Dominitz JA, et al. Guideline for the management of ingested foreign bodies. *Gastrointest Endosc.* 2002;55:802-806.
2. Hachimi-Idrissi S, Corne L, Vandenplas Y. Management of ingested foreign bodies in childhood: our experience and review of the literature. *Eur J Emerg Med.* 1998;5:319-323.
3. Blaho KE, Merigian KS, Winbery SL, et al. Foreign body ingestions in the emergency department: case reports and review of treatment. *J Emerg Med.* 1998;16:21-26.
4. Kamal I, Thompson J, Paquette DM. The hazards of vinyl glove ingestion in the mentally retarded patient with pica: new implications for surgical management. *Can J Surg.* 1999;42:201-204.
5. McKechnie JC. Gastroscopic removal of a phytobezoar. *Gastroenterology.* 1972;62:1047-1051.
6. Webb WA. Management of foreign bodies of the upper gastrointestinal tract: update. *Gastrointest Endosc.* 1995;41:39-51.

7. Li ZS, Sun ZX, Zou DW, et al. Endoscopic management of foreign bodies in the upper-GI tract: experience with 1088 cases in China. *Gastrointest Endosc.* 2006;64:485-492.

8. Velitchkov NG, Grigorov GI, Losanoff JE, et al. Ingested foreign bodies of the gastrointestinal tract: retrospective analysis of 542 cases. *World J Surg.* 1996;20:1001-1005.

9. Silva RG, Ahluwalia JP. Asymptomatic esophageal perforation after foreign body ingestion. *Gastrointest Endosc.* 2005;61:615-619.

I Was Washing and Suctioning to Get a Good Look at the Gastroesophageal Junction Varices and They Started to Bleed. I Could Not See Where the Bleeding Came From. What Should I Do?

John S. Goff, MD

This is not an uncommon situation. It is often encountered when we are performing endoscopy on patients with varices. It does, however, present an interesting dilemma as to what to do next. Obviously, you now need to consider what options are available to stop an acute bleed of major proportion from varices in the distal esophagus. The main options available are balloon tamponade (Sengstaken-Blakemore tube preferably with the Minnesota modification), medical therapy with agents that lower portal pressure (nitrates, beta blockers, vasopressin, and octreotide), endoscopic sclerotherapy, endoscopic variceal ligation, or some combination of these. Surgical intervention is rarely done these days due to generalized lack of experience. You could consider emergent placement of a transjugular intrahepatic portocaval shunt (TIPS), if available.

Octreotide given as a 50 mcg IV bolus followed by an infusion of 50 to 100 mcg/hr is currently the treatment of choice due to its rapid onset of action, minimal side effects, and efficacy. This should be initiated immediately.

Balloon tamponade is an effective means for temporarily controlling bleeding esophageal and cardia varices but is often only temporary; it is associated with several potential complications even if positioned correctly and requires some skill in placement. This should be used if endoscopic measures have already failed or there is no one with endoscopic experience available to try to stop the bleeding.

Endoscopic sclerotherapy has been used for many years to treat acute variceal bleeding, but the problem is that during massive bleeding, the site for injection may not be readily visible. It is extremely important to inject the sclerosant into the varices directly to avoid esophageal tissue damage and/or the development of mediastinitis and to achieve maximum benefit. There is literature on perivariceal injection of sclerosant, but the individual injected volumes used are usually small. The preferred method is to inject 1 to 2 ml of sclerosant (usually 5% ethanolamine oleate or sodium morrhuate 50 mg/ml in the United States) directly into the bleeding varix and then into the neighboring varices. The risk during heavy active bleeding with poor visibility is injecting a larger volume into one area, which can then result in tissue damage that will be a major problem a few days later.

Your best approach to this situation is to perform endoscopic variceal ligation (banding). This can easily be done even when the view is moderately hampered by blood. The patient's bed should be positioned so the head is up and the feet are down to facilitate flow into the stomach of the esophageal blood. If the patient is not able to protect his or her airway due to encephalopathy, you should consider tracheal intubation before proceeding. Tracheal intubation should also be considered if the patient is difficult to sedate lightly and will thus need deep sedation to achieve an adequate degree of calmness for the procedure.

For ligation, the multiple band device (Cook Medical, Bloomington, IN) is affixed to the end of a standard endoscope (they do not fit as well on the end of a therapeutic endoscope) and the patient is reintubated. You only need to know where the gastroesophageal junction is located to begin treatment. Aspirating blood from the esophagus with the banding device in place is possible, but it may foul the chamber at the end of the endoscope created by the banding device, which will make any attempt at banding futile. A flush using the needle provided in the banding kit via the biopsy port can remove clots from the banding device. Once you identify the gastroesophageal junction, bands are applied sequentially in a circular fashion moving up the esophagus. It is not imperative that the bands land directly on the varix, as banding mucosa without a varix has no adverse consequence. Usually, after applying a band or two, the field of view will start to be clearer due to decreased bleeding. This will allow you to do more directed band application to varices in the lower one-third of the esophagus. If the bleeding site should be visible when the banding device is on the endoscope, you should try to put a band directly over the spurting site. Bands can be applied at virtually any level in the esophagus without causing problems, but in the acute bleeder as described they usually do not need to be above the lower one-third. After this initial banding, the next session should be in 7 to 10 days to avoid rebleeding. Subsequent sessions are from 2 to 4 weeks until the varices are ablated.

References

1. Hunt PS, Korman MG, Hansky J, Parkin WG. An 8-year prospective experience with balloon tamponade in the control of bleeding esophageal varices. *Dig Dis Sci*. 1982;27:414-416.
2. Sanowski RA, Waring JP. Endoscopic techniques and complications in variceal sclerotherapy. *J Clin Gastroenterol*. 1987;9:504-513.
3. Stiegmann GV, Goff JS, Michaletz-Onody PA, et al. Endoscopic sclerotherapy as compared with endoscopic ligation for bleeding esophageal varices. *N Engl J Med*. 1987;326:1527-1532.

WHAT IS THE CURRENT RECOMMENDATION FOR ENDOSCOPIC SURVEILLANCE OF BARRETT'S ESOPHAGUS, AND HOW CAN WE IMPROVE THE RESULTS WITH THE CURRENT TECHNOLOGIES?

Paulo Sakai, MD, PhD, and Fauze Maluf-Filho, MD

A number of observational studies have suggested that patients with Barrett's esophagus (BE) in whom adenocarcinoma was detected in a surveillance program have their lesions at an earlier stage. The 5-year survival rate has been improved, compared to patients not undergoing routine endoscopic surveillance.[1] Therefore, current practice guidelines recommend endoscopic surveillance of patients with BE in an attempt to detect cancer at an early and potentially curable stage.

A cellular atypia confined to the epithelium is called dysplasia and is considered as a histological marker for the development of invasive adenocarcinoma in BE. According to the American Society for Gastrointestinal Endoscopy (ASGE) guideline,[2] for patients with established BE of any length and with no dysplasia, after 2 consecutive examinations within 1 year, an acceptable interval for additional surveillance is at every 3 years. If the presence or degree of dysplasia is indeterminate and there is evidence of acute inflammation due to gastroesophageal acid reflux, repeat biopsy should be performed after 8 weeks of effective acid-suppression therapy. Surveillance in patients with low-grade dysplasia (LGD) is recommended and a follow-up esophagogastroduodenoscopy (EGD) (ie, at 6 months) should be performed with biopsies in the area of dysplasia. If LGD is confirmed, then one possible management scheme would be surveillance at 12 months and yearly thereafter as long as dysplasia persists. Patients with high-grade dysplasia (HGD)

Figure 8-1. (A) Endoscopic view of Barrett's esophagus using white light and (B) the same lesion examined with the NBI system.

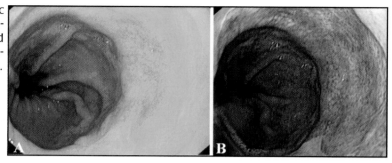

are at significant risk for prevalent or incidental cancer. HGD confirmed by two pathologists can be treated either by esophagectomy or by endoscopic management, which may consist of either endoscopic therapy or heightened surveillance. Patients who are surgical candidates may elect to have definitive therapy. Patients who elect surveillance endoscopy should undergo follow-up every 3 months for at least 1 year, with multiple biopsies obtained at 1 cm intervals. After 1 year of no cancer detection, the interval of surveillance may be lengthened if there are no dysplastic changes on 2 subsequent endoscopies performed at 3-month intervals. There is minor variation between societal recommendations regarding surveillance of HGD. The American College of Gastroenterology (ACG) guidelines recommend a repeat endoscopy with biopsies for patients in whom HGD is diagnosed; focal HGD (less than 5 crypts) can be followed by 3-month surveillance endoscopy, whereas endoscopic or surgical intervention is recommended for multifocal HGD.

Surveillance programs may become difficult in the general clinical practice and many clinicians may not even follow current practice guidelines. The strategy to perform a systematic jumbo biopsy protocol at 1 to 2 cm intervals plus biopsy of any mucosal abnormalities along the entire length of the BE has proved to miss cancer in patients with HGD. Using newer endoscopic techniques, we can target the biopsies to areas with higher probability of harboring dysplasia or cancer, improving the efficiency and sampling in surveillance programs. Techniques such as magnification endoscopy, chromoendoscopy with different stains, and instillation of 1.5% acetic acid have been examined and found to improve the accuracy of BE detection and early neoplasia compared with standard endoscopy in clinical trials.

Recently, narrow-band imaging (NBI) was developed, which is a special imaging technique that uses filter systems that allow passage of those spectral components of light, mainly blue color. This new endoscopic technique using high-definition television (HDTV) improves visualization and more details of mucosal surface and capillary system without the use of dyes (Figure 8-1). In several published studies, NBI in combination with magnification endoscopy seems to be a promising tool in the diagnosis of BE and abnormalities of structural surface patterns as well as irregular microvascular patterns, predicting dysplasia areas with high sensitivity and specificity.[3] One study compared NBI with high-resolution endoscopy in patients with known BE undergoing surveillance. The majority of HGD and early cancer could be detected by using chromoendoscopy and high-resolution endoscope alone with a statistically similar detection rate when compared with NBI alone.[4]

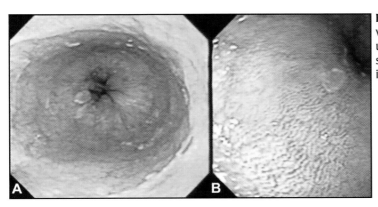

Figure 8-2. (A) Endoscopic view of Barrett's esophagus using a high-resolution endoscope and (B) the view after instillating 1.5% acetic acid.

The NBI technique is useful for BE surveillance, and the instillation of acetic acid on the mucosal surface can enhance the contrast, disclosing areas of subtle mucosal abnormalities in order to target biopsies. However, the use of high magnification with NBI may be confusing because the meaning of mucosal and vascular patterns demands a learning curve, and one single international classification would be desirable. In the future, this new generation of endoscope should be considered for routine use.

In clinical practice, the NBI system is not always available and we have recommended the use of high-resolution endoscope and 1.5% acetic acid instillation in the distal esophagus with BE, washing out with water after 2 minutes (Figure 8-2). A careful examination can disclose subtle mucosal abnormalities, such as ulceration, erosion, plaque, nodule, or other luminal irregularity in the Barrett's segment that should be biopsied.

References

1. Wang KK, Wongkeesong M, Buttar NS. American Gastroenterological Association technical review on the role of the gastroenterologist in the management of esophageal carcinoma. *Gastroenterology.* 2005;128:1471-1505.
2. ASGE guideline: the role of endoscopy in the surveillance of premalignant conditions of the upper GI tract. *Gastrointest Endosc.* 2006;63:570-580.
3. Goda K, Tajiri H, Ikegami M et al. Usefulness of magnifying endoscopy with narrow band imaging for the detection of specialized intestinal metaplasia in columnar-lined esophagus and Barrett's adenocarcinoma. *Gastrointest Endosc. 2007;65:36-46.*
4. Kara MA, Peters FP, Rosmolen WD, et al. High-resolution endoscopy plus chromoendoscopy or narrow-band imaging in Barrett's esophagus: a prospective randomized crossover study. *Endoscopy. 2005;37:929-936.*

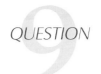
YOU WERE CALLED BY THE ER PHYSICIAN REGARDING A WOMAN WHO ATTEMPTED TO COMMIT SUICIDE BY DRINKING SOME "TOILET CLEANING SOLUTION." THERE WERE OBVIOUS BURNS AROUND THE MOUTH AND TONGUE. WHAT WOULD YOU DO NEXT?

Rajesh Gupta, MD, DM, and D. Nageshwar Reddy, MD, DM, FRCP, DSc

Ingestion of a corrosive substance is a common medical emergency. In adults, it is generally deliberate with suicidal intent. The first task while attending such a patient is to assess the hemodynamic stability of the patient. Whenever respiratory symptoms are present, the airway must be secured either by endotracheal intubation or tracheostomy. Once the patient is stable hemodynamically, the detailed history and physical examination is performed. There is poor corelation between symptoms and extent of injury. Many patients are asymptomatic initially and the symptoms may be delayed for several hours. After examination and lab investigations, chest and upright abdominal radiographs are advised. If radiographs are negative for signs perforation and clinical suspicion is high, water soluble contrast enhanced computed tomography (CT) of the chest or abdomen is advised.[1,2] Several studies have documented the efficacy and safety of early esophagogastroduodenoscopy (EGD) in corrosive-induced GI injuries. Early EGD assesses not only the grade of injury but helps in planning further management.[3] The patients with normal EGD, comprising about 40% to 80% of patients, can be safely discharged. Those with grade I and grade IIa injuries (edema, erythema, erosions, and on circumferential ulcers) can be started on a liquid diet and can be discharged after observation of 48 to 72 hours. Patients with grade IIb and III injuries (circumferential ulcers—multiple deep ulcers with brown, black, or grey discoloration) need close monitoring for the next 2 to 3 days, as the possibility of short- and long-term complications is very high. Of this group of patients, 70% to 100% develop strictures. Patients with grade IV injury need emergency surgery.[4] EGD is not recommended if the patient has evidence of perforation or delayed presentation (more than 7 days) after corrosive ingestion.

Animal studies have shown that immediate neutralization (within 30 minutes) of corrosive substance may reduce the extent of injury. However, this apparent benefit has not been proved in human studies. In fact, many experts believe that heat produced during neutralization reaction may exacerbate the extent of injury. As a policy in our institute, we do not recommend the use of neutralizing agents or emetics. There is no evidence to suggest that glucocorticoids prevent stricture formation. In fact, the administration of glucocorticoids may mask the signs of peritonitis or mediastinitis and increase the risk of infection. Hence the use of steroids is not recommended. There are no studies to suggest the beneficial effect of the prophylactic use of antibiotics. Most experts recommend that antibiotics should be used only if there is a specific indication. Nutrition is an important issue in patients with acute corrosive injuries. Oral feeding can be started early if EGD, is normal or shows grade I or grade IIA injuries. If the patient is unable to swallow or perforation is suspected, then parenteral nutrition is advised. There is no data to suggest that oral feeding is injurious in acute corrosive injuries. A nasogastric tube insertion for enteral feeding may be used if oral feeds are not tolerated. We prefer feeding jejunostomy if the patient continues to have severe odynophagia or absolute dysphagia. The role of early dilatation in acute corrosive injuries is controversial. There are no data to suggest that early dilatation prevents esophageal stricture. On the contrary, early dilatation increases the risk of complications and may accelerate fibrosis and stricture formation. We recommend dilatation of strictures after 4 to 6 weeks of corrosive injury. The role retrievable self-expanding metal stent (SEMS) in corrosive stricture is under evaluation and seems to be promising. In our center, we had good results with retrievable SEMS in tight corrosive strictures. Because the ingestion of corrosive agents in adults is usually suicidal, psychiatric evaluation and counseling is advised after discharge.

References

1. Kikendall JW. Caustic ingestion injuries. *Gastroenterol Clin North Am.* 1991;20:847.
2. Cellor JP, Fogel RP, Boland R. Liquid caustic ingestion spectrum of injury. *Arch Intern Med.* 1980;140:501.
3. Zargar SA, Kochhar R, Nagi B, et al. The role of fiberoptic endoscopy in the management of corrosive ingestion and modified endoscopic classification of burns. *Gastrointest Endosc.* 1991;37:65.
4. Estrera A, Taylor W, Mills LJ, Platt MR. Corrosive burns of the oesophagus and stomach: a recommendation for an aggressive surgical approach. *Ann Thorac Surg.* 1986;41:276.

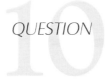
WHAT IS THE BEST TREATMENT FOR DUODENAL OR AMPULLARY ADENOMA, AND WHAT IS THE CURRENT RECOMMENDATION FOR SURVEILLANCE AFTER TREATMENT?

Richard A. Kozarek, MD

Ampullary tumors historically presented late with jaundice, bleeding, relapsing pancreatitis, or duodenal obstruction and were treated with radical pancreaticoduodenectomy and, less commonly, transduodenal resection and dual sphincteroplasty. Endoscopy in this setting was limited diagnostically to tissue acquisition and therapeutically to biliary stent placement or sphincterotomy in high surgical risk patients with obstructive jaundice. Currently, the majority of adenomas are found incidentally during screening for reflux or dyspepsia or follow-up of C-loop adenomas in patients with Gardner's syndrome.

Earlier diagnosis allows the potential for endoscopic as opposed to surgical resection, but neither endoscopic papillectomy nor local tumor ablation should be considered in isolation.[1,2] If found, incidentally, multiple biopsies should be done to rule out malignancy or a tumor with unusual histology such as carcinoid (Figure 10-1). Symptomatic patients, in turn, invariably require an abdominal computed tomography (CT) scan and measurement of tumor markers to include CEA and CA 19-9. Assuming CT and biopsy fail to demonstrate malignancy, there have been a number attempts to define endoscopic nonresectability. The latter include extremely large (4 to 5 cm) lesions, an ulcerated papilla, lesions that extend laterally and encompass less than 30% to 50% of the duodenal lumen, and a hard lesion that fails to elevate with a submucosal injection.[3] Likewise, polyps that extend a significant length (0.5 to 1.0 cm) into the bile duct or pancreas as F by endoscopic retrograde cholangiopancreatography (ERCP) or magnetic resonance

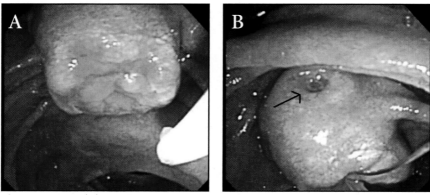

Figure 10-1. (A) Endoscopy demonstrates large ampullary adenoma (B) with fistula from tumor into bile duct (arrow).

Figure 10-2. Arrow delineates adenoma and copious air in biliary tree.

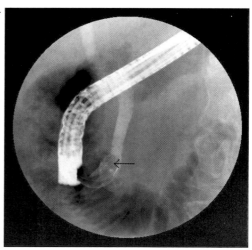

cholangiopancreatography (MRCP) are considered by many to be unresectable endoscopically (Figure 10-2). What role endoscopic ultrasound (EUS) or intraductal ultrasound (IDUS) plays in patients with ampullary adenomas is controversial. Some endoscopists believe that EUS should be undertaken in all patients with ampullary adenomas to preclude the risk of resection in patients with invasive malignancy. I use EUS infrequently and reserve it for patients in whom pancreas protocol CT fails to show malignancy but in whom local infiltration or the question of endoscopic resectability remains uncertain.

Technique

Technically, with the exception of asymptomatic and nonenlarging microadenomas of the papilla of Vater, which are virtually ubiquitous in Gardner's patients, ampullary adenomas should be treated. As noted above, historical treatment was usually done surgically, either with transduodenal papillectomy with concomitant sphincteroplasty or by means of Whipple procedure.

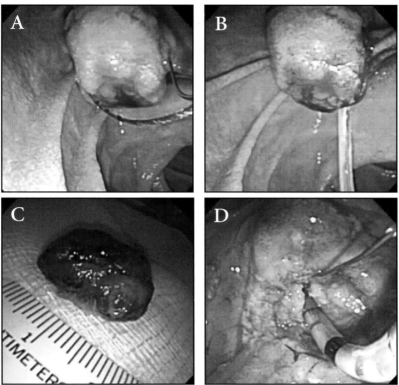

Figure 10-3. (A, B, C) Note papillectomy and (D) biliary sphincterotomy.

Endoscopic treatment of ampullary adenomas was initially limited to direct thermal ablation, most commonly with a Nd-YAG laser, but more recently with argon plasma coagulation (APC). Both treatment modalities have been associated with edematous obstruction of the pancreaticobiliary outlet with resultant jaundice, cholangitis, or obstructive pancreatitis. As a consequence, these modalities are currently used primarily to treat residual adenomatous tissue at the edge of a papillectomy site. Snare papillectomy, in turn, can be done in a piecemeal fashion for lesions less than 2 to 3 cm but can usually be done with a single resection using a blended current. I do an ERCP in all patients prior to resection, both to assure that there is no tumor growth into the pancreaticobiliary (PB) tree (see Figure 10-2) as well as to define landmarks to facilitate post-papillectomy PB drainage.[1] Some endoscopists utilize submucosal papilla injection to buffer the duodenal wall prior to resection as well as to define a non-"lifting sign" in the setting of infiltrating neoplasm. I do not. Such injections often blur tissue planes and require considerably more electrical current to facilitate transection of the papilla.

Following baseline ERCP and papillectomy, I undertake a biliary sphincterotomy using a blended or pulsed current and pancreatic sphincterotomy with pure cut current (Figure 10-3), placing stents in both ducts to protect against edematous obstruction of the duct orifices (Figure 10-4). APC treatment of the edges or small bleeding areas is sometimes required.

Data from a multicenter, retrospective series by Catalano et al[4] has noted a 17% incidence of pancreatitis in patients in whom no stent was inserted versus 3.3% of patients undergoing prophylactic pancreatic duct stenting. Moreover, subsequent stenosis of the PD sphincterotomy fell from 18.4% of patients to 1.1% in patients who had prophylactic

Figure 10-4. (A) Following guidewire placement into the pancreatic duct, (B) stents were placed into the pancreaticobiliary tree.

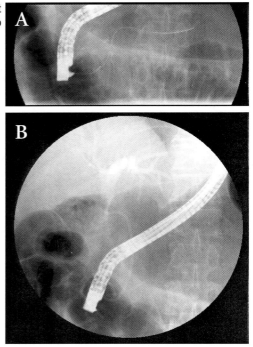

stenting. Although early and late biliary complications were comparable between patients who did or did not have biliary stenting, early bouts of cholangitis and cholestasis have changed my practice patterns to favor prosthesis placement in most patients.

Results

There are now numerous series that suggest that thermal ablation of the papilla is associated with a higher side-effect profile, less effective eradication of the ampullary adenoma, and need for significantly more interventions when compared to papillectomy. Moreover, there appears to be a 3- to 4-fold increased risk for ultimate development of malignancy when compared to papillectomy. As such, thermal ablation should play a big part in the treatment of ampullary adenomas, usually to "touch up" the margins of a resection site or to treat the adenomatous tissue (micro-adenomas) at the papillectomy site that frequently occur in Gardner's syndrome.

Han and Kim[5] have published a wonderful review of papillectomy. Currently, around 800 patients have been published in case reports, abstracts, and clinical series. Approximately one-quarter of patients have had Gardner's syndrome and three-quarters have had sporadic adenomas. Patients presented with jaundice, cholangitis, pancreatitis, weight loss, or chronic cholangitis, or more commonly, these were found during screening endoscopies. Lesions larger than 3 cm as well as patients with Gardner's adenomas were less likely to have long-term successful treatment, although 80% of total patients had long-term cure. Up to 10% of patients in some of the series were found to have underlying malignancy requiring definitive surgery. Procedural complications approximated 10%, most commonly bleeding or pancreatitis, and the perforation rate ranged between 0% and 3%. There was a single procedural mortality in this composite of patient series.

Follow-Up

Not only do patients with ampullary adenomas resected endoscopically need stent retrieval and papillectomy site inspection and biopsy at 4 to 6 weeks, they need long-term follow-up. Follow-up includes a baseline colonoscopy to assure that there are not concomitant colon adenomas as well as evaluation of the ampullectomy site with a side-viewing scope. Contingent upon the patient and the assumption of complete eradication of the ampullary adenoma, screening should occur at least yearly for the first 3 years and more frequently in patients with underlying genetic disorders.

In the review by Han and Kim,[5] a 15% recurrence rate was noted. This rate is a guesstimate, at best, as "recurrences" between 1 and 3 months post resection are much more likely related to incomplete resection than a true recurrence. Nevertheless, residual or recurrent disease is usually readily handled endoscopically and the recurrence rates are probably comparable to the 12.5% rates reported in patients undergoing open surgical transduodenal papillectomy for ampullary adenomas.

Although it is clear that endoscopic papillectomy has supplanted surgery in most patients with amenable lesions, it is also clear that there are lesions that are better handled surgically.[2] They include ulcerated or infiltrated lesions, patients who are found to have underlying malignancy in their resected specimens, Gardner's patients in whom the papilla may be only one of hundreds of large and enlarging C-loop adenomas, lesions extending a significant distance into the PB tree, and those in whom the adenoma encompasses a considerable circumferential component of the C-loop wall.

Figures 10-1 through 10-4 depict papillectomy in a high surgical risk patient who had significant dysplasia but no definite malignancy in his resected specimen.

References

1. Kozarek RA. Endoscopic resection of ampullary neoplasms. *J Gastrointest Surg.* 2004;8:932-934.
2. Tran TC, Vitale GC. Ampullary tumors: endoscopic versus operative management. Review. *Surg Innov.* 2004;11:255-263.
3. Kahaleh M, Shami VM, Brock A, et al. Factors predictive of malignancy and endoscopic resectability in ampullary neoplasia. *Am J Gastroenterol.* 2004;99:2335-2339.
4. Catalano MF, Linder JD, Chak A, et al. Endoscopic management of adenoma of the major duodenal papilla. *Gastrointest Endosc.* 2004;59:225-232.
5. Han J, Kim MH. Endoscopic papillectomy for adenomas of the major duodenal papilla (with video). Review. *Gastrointest Endosc.* 2006;63:292-301.

WHAT SHOULD I DO IF I HAVE INADVERTENTLY PERFORATED THE VISCUS DURING AN ENDOSCOPY?

Gregory Haber, MD

Anticipating higher-risk procedures should prepare the endoscopist for appropriate management and a game plan if a perforation actually occurs. High-risk procedures would include the following:

1. Esophagoscopy with a history of dysphagia, especially transfer dysphagia as occurs with a Zenker's diverticulum, or a known stricture

2. Large paraesophageal hernia

3. Prior radiation

4. Anastomotic narrowing

5. Altered anatomy as with colonic interposition, Billroth II, Roux-en-Y anastomoses, or hepatico and pancreatico jejunostomy

6. Use of an oblique or side-viewing endoscope, as with echoendoscopes or duodenoscopes when forward visualization is limited

7. Presence of luminal content such as ingested material, blood, or fluid that obscures the desired orifice

8. Large balloon dilation as for achalasia

9. Endoscopic mucosal resection or submucosal dissection of flat lesions or submucosal tumors

If a high-risk situation is known, the scheduling of the procedure should not be at the end of the day or after hours, when the radiologic or surgical backup may not be readily available. Contacting the supportive services in advance to be on hand or to consult the patient in preparation for alternative management is prudent. As always, consideration of a referral to a center of expertise is an option if your experience with the high-risk procedure is limited or if the necessary backup is not available in your institution. Likewise, a Friday procedure is not ideal because follow-up on a weekend is less desirable.

Recognition

Part of recognition is having the tactile sense of the tension being exerted on the wall of the gut. This is particularly relevant when advancing around sharp angulations in the gut. Examples follow:

1. Gastrojejunostomy especially entering the afferent limb, which has a more angulated take off with short afferent limbs in retro colic anastomoses
2. Enteroscopy with a history of prior surgery or adhesions
3. Diverticular disease with tethered sigmoid loops
4. Advancing from the hepatico or choledoch jejunostomy to the pancreatico jejunostomy within a short fixed loop of jejunum
5. Traversing the ligament of Treitz either in a prograde or retrograde direction
6. Reversing direction in an enteroenterostomy

Sensing the force being exerted on the wall of the gut is of paramount importance in prevention of perforation. That requires minimizing the resistance at the level of the mouth by ensuring adequate lubrication around the mouth guard and on the shaft of the scope. If an overtube is being used, similarly the scope should be well lubricated and the overtube irrigated as needed for hydrophilic linings. If working with a trainee or if asked to assist another endoscopist, when first taking over the procedure, the scope should be withdrawn from the point where the endoscopist is stuck back to a relatively straight position so as to appreciate the variability in resistance in reaching the level of obstruction to passage.

The mucosal lining creates a "red out" when the lens of the scope is flush against the wall at difficult turns, and therefore, when no luminal view is available, at least the sliding of the mucosa must be appreciated as the scope is advanced. If the view is lost due to mucus or foreign material, a water flush may help and serves to lubricate the mucosa for easier sliding of the scope tip along the wall. Once blanching of the mucosa occurs, the scope needs to be withdrawn but in a very slow manner, as there may be a paradoxic forward force due to unlooping along the shaft when this is done.

A perforation can be caused by the tip of the scope rupturing the gut wall or a bend in the shaft of the scope tearing the wall, usually in a longitudinal fashion. When a perforation by the tip occurs, there is initially a loss of view as the scope is in the wall. At times, due to the increased resistance at the level of the muscularis propria, there may be time to withdraw, leaving a mucosal tear only and aborting before perforating.

The view after a perforation depends on the level of the perforation as one enters the retropharyngeal space, the mediastinum, peritoneal cavity, retroperitoneum, or retrorectal space. Entry into the peritoneal cavity is easily recognized, as the organs such as liver or gut are seen. However, this may not occur when the mesenteric border of the gut is traversed because only the fat may be seen. If there are adhesions, which is often the case because prior surgery is a risk factor, dissection of the fibrous tissue associated with these may appear like "candy floss." There may be little to see if blood or tissue obscures the lens. When entering the retroperitoneum, a loss of view also occurs, and it is important not to push forward without a luminal view. There may be less resistance to advancement after the intial perforation, which may give a false sense of security that the scope has finally traversed a difficult turn when in fact one may be pushing through the mediastinum or neck parallel to the true lumen. Once again, irrigation with water and withdrawal to obtain a better view is mandatory.

Management

Initial management of perforations no longer dictates an immediate call to the surgeon but rather an assessment as to the size, location, and whether it may be remediable with endoscopic tools. Part of this assessment relates to the clinical indication. For example, if an anastomotic stricture for the index procedure is likely to require multiple dilations and a perforation occurs early on, this may tip the scales in favor of surgery for the immediate complication as well as for definitive therapy of the underlying problem.

A perforation above the level of the upper esophageal sphincter (eg, through the valecular fossa or a Zenker's diverticulum) is always due to the scope tip. This area is difficult to evaluate as there are pharyngeal contractions and gagging. The best way to assess this is with a clear cap on the scope to splay apart the folds for better visualization. If access and orientation allow an adequate field of view, clips with small stems (ie, < 5 mm) may be applied, especially in a diverticulum. Conservative measures include placement of a nasogastric tube under endoscopic vision so as not to inadvertently advance the tube when it is lodged in the mouth of the perforation. Antibiotics and acid suppression are routinely given for any perforation in the upper GI tract. Unfortunately, only a minority of these perforations is suitable for endoscopic management, and most require surgery with a transcervical drain.

Perforations along the body of the esophagus allow for better viewing and access, whereas at the gastroesophageal junction, the sphincter and puckering of folds may obscure the view of the perforation. Once again, a large friction cap on the scope tip such as a 16-mm oblique Olympus cap should open up the area for suitable inspection. In the esophagus, in addition to clip closure, there is the option of a covered metal or a solid plastic stent to bridge the perforation and prevent food and salivary contamination of the mediastinum. Stent options include covered metal stents such as the ultra flex or Alveolus (Alveolus Inc., Charlotte, NC) or a solid plastic polyflex stent. Unfortunately, migration is a major drawback, and attempts to secure the stent include clipping of the upper stent wire to the esophageal wall or tying a suture line to the top of the stent, which is then brought out through the nose and secured for a few days to try to allow the stent to become embedded with a hyperplastic inflammatory reaction around the stent.

The concern regarding endoscopic therapies is that if they do not succeed, the outcomes of delayed surgery are generally worse compared to early operation. After endoscopic measures, a limited radiologic exam with barium is useful to assess the effectiveness of the treatment in preventing a leak. If the patient is clinically stable with a minimal leak on radiographic studies in the first 12 hours, ongoing conservative treatment can continue.

A white blood cell (WBC) count less than 15,000 and a temperature less than 99° Celsius can be expected in the first 24 to 48 hours but should improve thereafter if the endoscopic therapy is adequate.

When the perforation involves the stomach, jejunum, ileum, or colon with a punched out hole into the peritoneal cavity, in addition to mechanical closure of the hole with clips, the pneumoperitoneum may cause respiratory distress and needs to be dealt with as well. Placement of clips should begin at the ends of the torn tissue because frequently the 12- to 14-mm wingspan of most clips will not span the defect in the middle. Working from the ends of the tear with aspiration to reduce distention should allow apposition of the opposing walls of the torn tissue.

If the bowel lumen collapses due to air loss into the peritoneal cavity, the position of the patient may be changed to elevate the area of the perforation so that the air tends to remain in that part of the bowel. As air is absorbed slowly and is irritating to the peritoneal lining, air insufflation should immediately be exchanged for carbon dioxide if it is available. In addition, large amounts of air in the peritoneal cavity may impair diaphragmatic movement, and decompression using a simple 16 or 18 Fr angiocath sleeve can bring about immediate relief. One can expect mild degrees of peritoneal irritation, but if frank peritonitis occurs, surgical intervention will be necessary. When the endoscopic therapy is adequate, there may be a low grade fever or mild leukocytosis, but the patient should not be tachycardic or toxic and should maintain bowel sounds.

If the tear occurs at an anastomotic site, the narrowed stricture lumen may be tight enough to hold a covered stent in place a sufficient time to allow healing. Conservative measures are more successful when there are adhesions and adherent loops of bowel that tend to localize the spillage from the perforation and may spontaneously wall off the area. The same is true with retroperitoneal perforations in the duodenal sweep or rectum. The lack of free peritoneal air reduces the clinical impact and improves the chance for definitive endoscopic treatment.

With larger perforations, as can occur with endoscopic submucosal dissection or use of a cap to suck the tissue prior to snare resection, loops have been used with limited success to entrap the folds around the perforation and then cinch them together. One described method requires a double-channel endoscope. An endoloop is passed down one channel and through the second channel; clips are deployed over the loop to secure the loop to the margins of the perforation. The arms of the closed clips should have enough space between them to allow movement of the loop, and as the loop is tightened, the tissue folds are drawn together with the clips, securing the tissue to the loop. Another approach has been the use of mesentery to fill the gap of the perforation and then clipping the margins of the perforated wall to the mesentery. This requires a grasping forceps to pull the mesentery into the hole of the perforation and then applying multiple clips around the circumference to hold the mesentery in place.

Conclusion

The presence of air in the peritoneal cavity no longer needs to be considered the clarion call for surgical intervention. With increasing frequency, in appropriately selected patients and perforations, endoscopic therapy and associated supportive measures can provide definitive treatment.

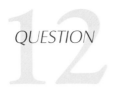
Is Fluoroscopy Absolutely Necessary for Dilation of Esophageal Stricture and Placement of Esophageal Stent?

Terry L. Jue, MD, and Walter Trudeau, MD

Esophageal stents palliate dysphagia caused by malignant esophageal strictures. The strictures may be due to cancer in the lumen or to extrinsic compression of the esophagus by adjacent tumors. A stent keeps the esophagus patent and allows patients to maintain oral intake and alimentary nutrition. The self-expanding metal stent (SEMS) was introduced in the 1990s and is now the most commonly used stent for palliating malignant esophageal strictures. Prior to placing a SEMS, an endoscopist will frequently dilate a malignant stricture in order to successfully deploy the stent across the site of narrowing. Fluoroscopy aids with dilation and positioning of the SEMS before deployment but is not always necessary. We will describe how to dilate an esophageal stricture and place a SEMS in the esophagus without fluoroscopy. The data supporting the use of removable, self-expanding plastic stents to treat benign strictures is limited, so we will focus on the use of a SEMS for palliating a malignant esophageal stricture.

A SEMS consists of a mesh of intertwined metal woven into a hollow tube. Manufacturers package stents in a compact form, where the stent is compressed tightly onto a deployment device designed to release the stent in the esophagus. Upon deployment, a SEMS expands radially and slowly begins to assume its intended shape. The expansile property maintains patency of the lumen across a stricture, and the woven mesh enables flexibility and conformation of the stent within the esophagus. After deployment, a SEMS exerts expansive pressure on the epithelium of the esophagus, inducing tissue reaction and growth. The reactive tissue grows into the mesh of the stent, securing the stent and reducing the likelihood of migration. A SEMS may have a proximal flange, which is a flared collar on the end of the stent designed to anchor and thus prevent migration. A SEMS may also be covered with an internal, impermeable lining. The covering prevents SEMS occlusion resulting from tumor growth between the wire mesh of a stent. The risk of migration in covered stents can be higher if the covering interferes with tissue anchoring that occurs when the stent expands and induces epithelial growth into its wire mesh.

Most endoscopists use fluoroscopy to deploy a SEMS at the correct location. Flouroscopy aids in placement because many deployment devices are too large to allow for endoscopic viewing during release. A SEMS has radiopaque markers on its deployment device that define each end of the stent under fluoroscopy. Manufacturers have designed esophageal stents with small-diameter delivery systems that allow you to place an endoscope in the esophagus alongside the unreleased stent. The delivery systems are 5 to 7 mm in diameter. With endoscopic viewing, you can see where the SEMS is relative to the proximal end of a stricture and reposition if necessary before deployment. Many endoscopists use the direct-visualization feature of small-diameter delivery system SEMS together with fluoroscopy. Studies demonstrate, however, that dilation of esophageal strictures and subsequent placement of a SEMS can be performed safely by endoscopy alone.[1-5]

When considering placement of a SEMS for a malignant esophageal stricture, determine whether an esophagram was performed. An esophagram can help determine the location, length, and extent of narrowing of the stricture. Endoscopy should be performed to measure the narrowing and the length of the stricture. Successful placement of a SEMS requires the stricture to be at least 13 mm in diameter. Oftentimes, a malignant stricture in a patient with dysphagia is less than 13 mm across. If so, dilation should be performed to 13 mm before placing a SEMS.

Strictures can be dilated using either bougies or through-the-scope radially expansive balloons. Both bougies and balloons require a guidewire for proper positioning. We prefer a stiff 0.035 Cook Endoscopy Savary (Cook Endoscopy, Inc, Winston-Salem, NC) guidewire for bougie dilation and stent deployment. A balloon usually comes with its own guidewire. If the stricture can be traversed by the endoscope, then the guidewire can be placed through the channel of the scope and left in the antrum. If the stricture cannot be passed by the scope, then the guidewire can be passed through the channel of the scope, gently through the stricture, and into the stomach. Pay attention to the wire markings that correspond to the distance advanced so you know when the wire is in the distal stomach.

When the stricture is tortuous or unpassable endoscopically, we prefer to avoid bougie dilation. A tortuous stricture may deflect the tip of the bougie into the wall of the esophagus, causing perforation. Dilation of a stricture whose proximal end cannot be passed by the scope can be performed with a balloon first. If the stricture is long but not tortuous, bougie dilation can be performed after initial dilation. If the stricture is short, then using the same balloon again for distal dilation is adequate.

For tumors in the esophagus, we recommend using a covered stent and placing the covering across the tumor. When choosing the length of the stent, keep in mind the length of the stricture and the location. With strictures of the upper esophagus, be sure the proximal end of the stent will not be at or above the cricopharyngeus muscle. A stent across the upper esophageal sphincter could cause aspiration and even tracheal compression. Avoid placing a stent for strictures of the lower esophagus too far into the stomach because the stent can impact against the posterior wall and cause ulceration.

The use of fluoroscopy in placing an esophageal stent relies primarily upon establishing a radiopaque mark to define the distal end of the stricture. A way to establish the mark

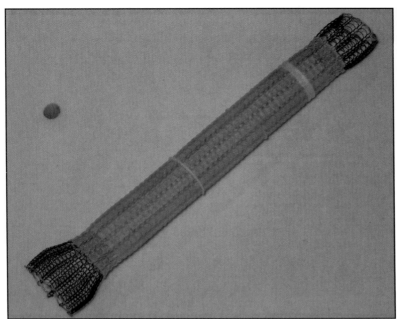

Figure 12-1. The Ultraflex stent (from Boston Scientific) showing the membrane covered shaft of the stent and the uncovered mesh on either ends.

is by advancing the tip of the endoscope to the distal end of the stricture and taping a coin on the body surface at a site corresponding fluoroscopically with the endoscope tip. A spot film is taken with fluoroscopy, and the marker is repositioned until matching with the tip of the endoscope. The use of an external marker can become inaccurate because of the patient's respiratory movements, known as the "parallax effect". An approach to establish the distal end of the stricture without parallax is by the submucosal injection of contrast. Unfortunately, this method is prone to inaccuracy because the contrast can diffuse into the submucosal tissue plane and fade radiographically. We prefer endoscopic placement of a metal clip just distal to the stricture to create a marker unaffected by parallax. For strictures at the gastroesophageal junction, however, placement of the clip in the proximal stomach can be challenging, as retroflexion of the endoscope is usually necessary.

A SEMS with a small-diameter deployment device can be placed across a malignant esophageal stricture by endoscopy without the use of flouroscopy. After the SEMS is advanced over a guidewire, you can introduce the endoscope into the esophagus and directly visualize where the proximal end of the stent lies relative to the stricture. After deployment, you may carefully advance the endoscope to ensure patency across the stricture. Gentle withdrawal of the endoscope out of the stent avoids displacement.

In the United States, the Boston Scientific (Natick, MA) Ultraflex esophageal stent location is the only commercially available SEMS with multiple published articles describing large numbers of patients who underwent successful placement of the stent without fluoroscopy.[2,3,5] The Ultraflex is covered across its central portion, with a proximal uncovered flange and distal uncovered segment (Figure 12-1). An esophageal covered SEMS should be at least 5 cm longer than the stricture to ensure the covered portion of the stent is across the tumor. Two outer radiopaque markers on the delivery system indicate the ends of the SEMS after deployment (Figure 12-2). Two inner radiopaque markers represent the borders of the covered portion of the SEMS after deployment (Figure 12-2). Hence, the

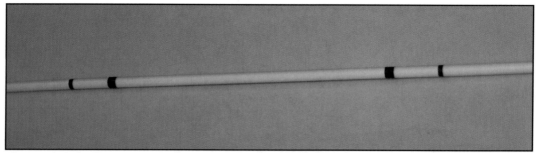

Figure 12-2. Radiopaque markers indicating the length of the covered stent help positioning of the stent through the esophageal obstruction before stent deployment.

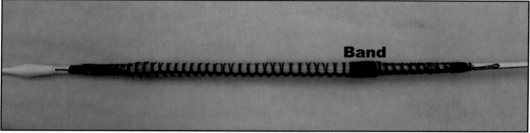

Figure 12-3. Proximal release Ultraflex stent. The "band" indicates the position of the proximal end of the stent, and this visual marker helps with positioning of the stent during deployment even without fluoroscopy.

proximal inner marker should be above the beginning of the stricture and the distal inner marker below the distal end of the stricture.

The Ultraflex stent is designed with either a proximal or distal release mechanism. We prefer the proximal release system when placing the stent without fluoroscopy. The proximal release covered stent has a band of tight threading on its proximal end (Figure 12-3). The midpoint of this band represents the location of the proximal end of the stent after release. We use the band as a visual aid to position the SEMS. Since the uncovered and flared part of the stent is 1.5 cm long after deployment, and the midpoint of the band represents the proximal end of the SEMS, we create a mark on the stent 3 cm distal to the middle of the band. With the aid of endoscopy, we line up our created mark with the proximal end of the stricture. The SEMS is then ready for release. Our approach ensures that the covered part of the SEMS is across the tumor. The distal release Ultraflex stent does not have a band of threading, but you can visualize the outermost radiopaque mark (Figure 12-4) and then create a visible mark 3 cm distally. The created mark can then be placed at the edge of the stricture before deploying the stent. Studies have demonstrated the placement of distal-release Ultraflex stents without fluoroscopy.[3-5] Be mindful, however, that Boston Scientific only supports the placement of proximal Ultraflex stents without fluoroscopy.

Placing a SEMS by endoscopy alone saves the costs and time associated with arranging for fluoroscopy. However, always place the safety of the patient first and consider fluoroscopy with difficult strictures. Usually, though, an endoscopist can place a SEMS by direct visualization and effectively palliate dysphagia due to malignant strictures.

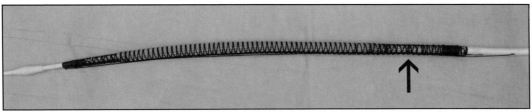

Figure 12-4. The distal release Ultraflex stent does not have the "band" as a visual marker and is preferably deployed with fluoroscopy control.

References

1. Wilkes EA, Jackson LM, Cole AT, et al. Insertion of expandable metallic stents in esophageal cancer without fluoroscopy is safe and effective: a 5-year experience. *Gastrointest Endosc.* 2007;65(6):923-929.
2. Ben Soussan E, Antonietti M, Lecleire S, et al. Palliative esophageal stent placement using endoscopic guidance without fluoroscopy. *Gastroenterol Clin Biol.* 2005;29(8-9):785-788.
3. Austin AS, Khan Z, Cole AT, Freeman JG. Placement of esophageal self-expanding metallic stents without fluoroscopy. *Gastrointest Endosc.* 2001;54(3):357-359.
4. Rathore OI, Coss A, Patchett SE, Mulcahy HE. Direct-vision stenting: the way forward for malignant oesophageal obstruction. *Endoscopy.* 2006;38(4):382-384.
5. White RE, Mungatana C, Topazian M. Esophageal stent placement without fluoroscopy. *Gastrointest Endosc.* 2001;53(3):348-351.

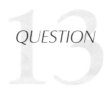

I Have a Patient With Advanced HIV and Severe Odynophagia. He Has Failed an Empiric Course of Fluconazole. What Agents Commonly Cause Odynophagia in This Population?

John P. Cello, MD

Dysphagia (difficulty in swallowing), odynophagia (painful deglutition) and esophagospasm (spontaneous nonswallowing substernal chest pain) are extremely common among patients with advanced human immunodeficiency virus (HIV) disease. Multiple etiologies may be found in these patients. Clearly the most common cause of esophageal difficulty of patients with acquired immune deficiency syndrome (AIDS) is *Candida albicans*, a common opportunistic fungal agent found in the gastrointestinal tract of all individuals. Well over 50% of patients with AIDS who complain of esophageal symptoms have *Candida* esophagitis. Most patients, but certainly not all, with *Candida* esophagitis have thrush, a white cheesy exudate on the tongue and soft palate. *Candida* esophagitis is so common that indeed the standard of care is for patients with AIDS and *any* esophageal complaints to treat through a full course of fluconazole. Fluconazole clearly controls *Candida* esophagitis and treats the acute infection but clearly does not eradicate *Candida*. Recurrence of *Candida* esophagitis is virtually universal in patients who are never rescued from a profound immunocompramised state.

Three other disease entities are encountered commonly in patients with severe immunosupression. These include cytomegalovirus, herpes simplex virus and idiopathic aphthous ulcers of the esophagus. The clinician must also be aware that noninfectious ulcerations may be found in a patient with AIDS, such as gastroesophageal reflux disease or pill esophagitis (occasionally related to nonsteroidal antiinflammatory drugs [NSAIDS], tetracycline or potassium chloride). Early infiltrating neoplasms of the gastroesophageal junction may likewise present with odynophagia as well as dysphagia. Uncommon causes of esophageal ulceration and odynophagia include histoplasmosis and even tuberculosis. The estimated frequencies of the principle disease entities in the esophagus are impressive. Roughly 20% to 50% of patients with HIV disease and any esophageal complaint are found to have *Candida* esophagitis. Cytomegalovirus (CMV) occurs in 10% to 15% of patients with odynophagia. Herpes simplex and idiopathic aphthous ulcers each account for between 5% and 15% of patients. Reflux esophagitis with esophageal ulcers occurs in 5% to 10% of patients. Endoscopically, it is possible to differentiate among these agents with a high degree of reliability, however endoscopic biopsies are mandatory. The endoscopic features together with biopsy are so reliable that very low threshold for endoscopy must be entertained in patients who fail to respond to an empiric course of fluconazole.

Most but not all patients with *Candida* esophagitis have thrush. Dysphagia is the most common clinical finding with relatively modest odynophagia. There is virtually no esophageal spasm or odynophagia in patients with *Candida* esophagitis and localization of the esophageal complaints on the anterior chest is poor since the infection is usually panesophageal but relatively superficial. The clinical features of cytomegalovirus esophagitis include minimal to moderate dysphagia but severe odynophagia and esophagospasm. The localization of esophageal complaints is fairly accurate. Herpes simplex esophagitis also has moderate dysphagia but severe odynophagia and esophagospasm. Its localization is also quite good. Aphthous idiopathic ulcers of the esophagus are similar to CMV in clinical presentation. Dysphagia is moderate, but odynophagia and esophagospasm are often severe with fair somatic localization.

The endoscopic features tend to be classic in these patients. There are a few patients who despite fluconazole treatment will have persistent *Candidasis*. While some of these patients are noncompliant, a few may have resistant *Candida* species such as *Candida tropicalis* or *Torulopsis glabrada*. Despite the finding of fairly classic elevated white plaques, patients who have failed fluconazole therapy should therefore be biopsied, not only the plaques themselves, but also the underlying mucosa. The biopsies should be submitted for fungal and viral cultures. Diagnosis of resistant *Candida* esophagitis must exclude other pathogens based upon histology and fungal culture. Response to therapy is excellent and in some patients who are fluconazole resistant other agents, including itraconazole, may be needed.

Cytomegalovirus esophagitis is characterized by very large deep "geographic" ulcers. The ulcers may be circumferential and of such length that virtually the entire esophagus is ulcerated. On occasion, the ulcers have undermined mucosa and sub mucosa, creating a false lumen. The diagnosis of CMV depends on histology with standard hematoxylin and eosin stains. The classic histologic feature is the presence of CMV infected endothelial cells. This is easily encountered on biopsy most of the time. Cultures are not helpful; in fact, they may be misleading. Many of the patients with advanced HIV disease have CMV viremia such that viral cultures are often positive. Response of CMV to ganciclovir or foscarnet is reasonably good.

Herpes simplex also produces ulcers of the esophagus; however, these ulcers are usually smaller but deeper and rarely are greater than 5 to 6 mm in diameter. The diagnosis is usually made by histology together with viral cultures. Response to acyclovir therapy

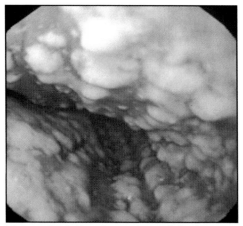

Figure 13-1. Esophageal candidiasis.

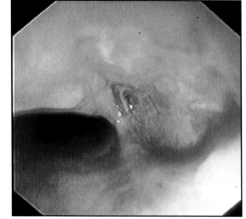

Figure 13-2. CMV ulcer.

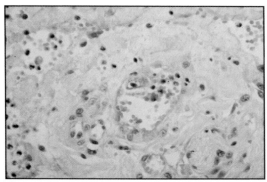

Figure 13-3. CMV endothelial cells.

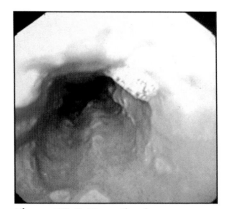

Figure 13-4. Herpetic ulcers.

is excellent. Idiopathic aphthous ulcers of the esophagus appear very similar to CMV ulcers. Idiopathic aphthous ulcers also are large, deep, nearly circumferential geographic ulcers. The diagnosis depends upon histology failing to demonstrate either CMV or herpes infected cells together with a negative viral culture. Therapy for idiopathic aphthous ulcers is distinctly different from the others since first line therapy usually includes thalidomide. Response to therapy is also quite good.

Figure 13-1 shows the classic endoscopic appearance of esophageal candidiasis with elevated white plaques extending virtually the entire length of the esophagus. Figure 13-2 shows the classic appearance of a CMV ulcer with an ulcer extending from the 12 o'clock to the 3 o'clock position on the slide. There is also a deeply penetrating sinus tract. The highest yield of biopsies for CMV is at the undermined margin or the ulcer base and Figure 13-3 shows CMV endothelial cells. Figure 13-4 shows herpetic ulcers, which are relatively small in size but may be relatively deep. Figure 13-5 shows classic herpes virus infected cells with Cowdry Type A inclusions. Figure 13-6 shows an idiopathic esophageal ulcer at the 6 to 8 o'clock position on the slide. This large geographic ulcer appears grossly similar to that of CMV. Only by biopsies with supplementary cultures can idiopathic aphthous ulcers be differentiated from CMV.

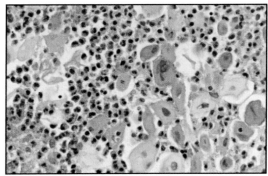

Figure 13-5. Herpes virus infected cells with Cowdry Type A inclusions.

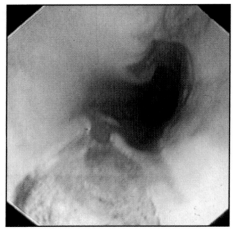

Figure 13-6. Idiopathic esophageal ulcer.

Occasionally, patients with advanced HIV disease have reflux esophagitis and ulcerations. The clinical suspicion of reflux esophagitis should be raised in individuals who have linear esophagitis and linear ulcerations radiating from the gastroesophageal junction above a hiatal hernia.

Performing an early endoscopy in patients with AIDS and esophageal symptoms is thus extremely beneficial, especially in patients who have failed empiric fluconazole therapy. Endoscopy with supplementary biopsies for histology and/or viral culture clearly allows the clinician to make a definitive diagnosis in most instances and promptly initiate specific therapy.

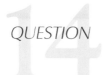
WHAT IS THE CURRENT EXPERT OPINION ON WHAT HEMOSTASIS TECHNIQUE TO USE IN TREATING A VISIBLE VESSEL OR DIEULAFOY LESION? WHEN SHOULD I INVOLVE A SURGEON?

Sanjay Hegde, MD, and Michael L. Kochman, MD, FACP

Advances in endoscopic therapy have greatly improved patient outcomes in the management of bleeding peptic ulcers and other upper gastrointestinal (UGI) arterial lesions. The prevalence of high risk stigmata of bleeding for patients with peptic ulcers is approximately 5% to 10% for active arterial spurting and 20% to 25% for nonbleeding visible vessels (Figure 14-1). The rebleeding rates for these lesions with medical therapy alone are 80% to 90% for active arterial spurting and 40% to 50% for visible vessels. Endoscopic therapy decreases these rebleeding rates to 18% and 10% to 15% respectively and can decrease blood transfusion requirements and hospital days.[1]

A variety of modalities are available for management of these lesions including thermal contact devices, mechanical hemostasis clips, and epinephrine injection. For initial diagnosis and treatment of suspected UGI bleeding, a therapeutic endoscope with a large suction channel is recommended. The mainstay of therapy for bleeding peptic ulcers is a combination of contact thermal therapy with epinephrine injection, which has been previously shown to be superior to epinephrine alone in achieving hemostasis with improvement in rebleeding rates, shorter hospital stay, and decreased need for operative intervention.[2]

Contact thermal devices include multipolar probes and heater probes. Multipolar probes achieve hemostasis by heating contacted tissue via passage of electrical current through the electrodes attached to the tip or sides of the tip of the probe. Resistance to

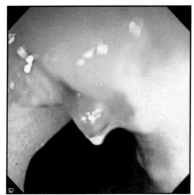

Figure 14-1. Gastric ulceration with visible vessel.

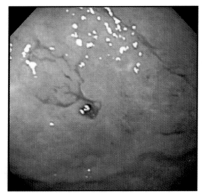

Figure 14-2. Gastric Dieulafoy lesion with oozing.

further coagulation occurs with increasing desiccation of coagulated tissue and thereby theoretically limits the depth of injury. Optimally, a 10 French probe is used and coagulation may be performed at 20 watts applied after initial irrigation of bleeding site. The duration of the therapy and the pulse frequency varies by report, but it is important that flattening of the bleeding lesion be achieved with the probe tip to cause coaptive thermal coagulation. Heater probes apply the energy by use of a ceramic tip which can heat more quickly. These are not limited in effect by tissue resistance and can achieve greater depth of coagulation; however, their use carries a higher risk of gastrointestinal perforation. For active arterial spurting, epinephrine injection (1:10,000 in normal saline) is applied in 0.5 to 1.0 mL aliquots in 4 quadrants along ulcer base prior to application of thermal contact therapy. For non-bleeding visible vessels, thermal contact therapy can be applied with epinephrine prior or after if bleeding occurs.

Mechanical hemostasis with hemoclips is also an effective treatment for arterial bleeding lesions. Hemoclips are steel grasping devices that are passed through the biopsy channel of the endoscope as part of a dedicated clip application system and achieve hemostasis via mechanical compression of a bleeding vessel. Early studies suggest that combination of thermal coagulation and epinephrine injection was superior to hemoclip application for achieving hemostasis.[3] Hemoclips can achieve effective hemostasis with or without adjunctive epinephrine injection.[4]

Dieulafoy lesions (exulceratio simplex, caliber persistent vessel) are rare lesions that account for approximately 1.9% of all patients with acute gastrointestinal hemorrhage. They are important as they often present with severe and recurrent bleeding. These lesions are characterized by presence of a relatively large artery in close proximity to the mucosal surface in the absence of mucosal ulceration (Figure 14-2). They are most commonly seen in the proximal stomach within 6 cm of the gastroesophageal (GE) junction along the lesser curvature of the stomach; however, they can be found throughout the gastrointestinal tract. Endoscopic criteria for diagnosis include 1) active arterial spurting or micropulsatile streaming from a < 3 mm mucosal defect (essentially the vessel itself), 2) visualization of a protruding vessel with or without active bleeding within a minute mucosal defect with normal surrounding mucosa, or 3) densely adherent clot with a narrow point of attachment to a minute mucosal defect or normal appearing mucosa, and the absence of ulceration. Endoscopic therapy is highly successful in treating these lesions, with hemostasis achieved in 96% of cases. Thermal contact therapy is the mainstay of treatment with epinephrine injection as a useful adjunct. Hemoclip application and endoscopic band ligation have also been applied to these lesions with good effect.[5]

Endoscopic therapy for bleeding ulcers and Dieulafoy lesions is very effective. Surgery is reserved for cases refractory to endoscopic hemostasis and for those in which rebleeding occurs and maximal endoscopic therapy has failed. It is advisable to have a surgeon involved in cases where initial endoscopic hemostasis is ineffective, the presentation itself was life-threatening, and in patients with high risk lesions that rebleed. Often endoscopic therapy is repeated before a definitive surgical or interventional radiology treatment in these cases.

References

1. Laine L, Peterson WL. Bleeding peptic ulcer. *N Engl J Med.* 1994;331(11):717-727.
2. Chung SSC, Lau JYW, Sung JJY, et al. Randomised comparison between adrenaline injection alone and adrenaline injection plus heat probe treatment for actively bleeding ulcers. *Brit Med J.* 1997;314(7090):1307.
3. Lin HJ, Hsieh Y, Tseng G, et al. A prospective, randomized trial of endoscopic hemoclip versus heater probe thermocoagulation for peptic ulcer bleeding. *Am J Gastroenterol.* 2002;97(9):2250-2254.
4. Saltzman JR, Strate LL, Di Sena V, et al. Prospective trial of endoscopic clips versus combination therapy in upper GI bleeding. *Am J Gastroenterol.* 2005;100(7):1503-1508.
5. Norton ID, Petersen BT, Sorbi D, et al. Management and long-term prognosis of Dieulafoy lesion. *Gastrointest Endosc.* 1999;50(6):762-767.

SECTION II

COLONOSCOPY

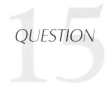
WHICH OF MY PATIENTS WITH ULCERATIVE COLITIS NEED "SURVEILLANCE" COLONOSCOPY? IF THEY ARE WELL MANAGED ON STABLE DOSES OF MEDICATION, WHY DO THEY NEED ELECTIVE COLONOSCOPY?

Francis A. Farraye, MD, MSc

Patients with long-standing ulcerative colitis are at an increased risk for developing dysplasia and colorectal carcinoma (CRC). This risk approaches 8% by 20 years and 18% by 30 years.[1] Recent data suggests that the risk of CRC in patients with ulcerative colitis may be lower than previously reported.[2] Patients with extensive Crohn's colitis also have an increased risk of CRC and should undergo regular surveillance.[3] At present, despite a lack of evidence from randomized controlled trials, surveillance colonoscopy is the best and most widely used method to detect dysplasia and cancer in inflammatory bowel disease (IBD) patients.[4-5]

A number of factors are associated with an increased risk of developing CRC in IBD.[4] These include a longer duration of colitis, greater extent of colonic involvement (no increase in proctitis patients, SIR 2.8 [CI: 1.6 to 4.4] in left sided ulcerative colitis (UC) and 14.8 [CI: 11.4 to 18.9] in pancolitis), family history of colorectal cancer (two-fold increase), primary sclerosing cholangitis, young age of IBD onset (some studies) and possibly backwash ileitis. A recent advance has been the appreciation that an increased severity of inflammation identified endoscopically and histologically is associated with cancer risk.[6] Using these clinical factors patients at an increased risk of developing dysplasia and/or CRC can be identified. Endoscopic findings may also help in the stratification of patients at highest risk of developing dysplasia or cancer. In a recent study, the presence of strictures (OR 4.62; CI 1.03 to 20.8) and pseudopolyps (OR 2.29; CI 1.28 to 4.11) were both predictors for the development of CRC on multivariate analysis.[7]

Table 15-1

Suggested **Performance** of Surveillance Colonoscopy

- Beginning approximately 7 to 8 years from the onset of colitis, all patients with UC should undergo an initial screening colonoscopy to determine the extent of colitis and check for neoplasia.
- Patients with left-sided colitis should follow the same schedule as those with extensive colitis, although some authorities suggest that regular surveillance for left-sided colitis should begin after 15 years of disease when the risk rises to that of extensive colitis.
- In the case of patients with primary sclerosing cholangitis, screening colonoscopy should be carried out at the time the biliary tract disease is diagnosed.
- If no dysplasia is detected, patients with extensive colitis (proximal to the hepatic flexure) should have repeat examinations every 1 to 2 years.
- If indefinite dysplasia is reported, the nature of the uncertainty should be ascertained from the pathologist. If the suspicion of dysplasia is high (ie, probably positive), short-term rebiopsy within 3 to 6 months or less may be indicated; if low (ie, probably negative), the interval should be reduced to every 6 to 12 months.
- Obtain 4 biopsy specimens of flat mucosa every 10 cm (consider sampling every 5 cm in the rectosigmoid).
- Place each quadruplicate set in a separate specimen jar (as opposed to pooling biopsy specimens from several colonic segments).
- Sample suspicious lesions or polyps.
- Make sure to biopsy flat mucosa around the base of any suspicious polyp and submit specimen in a separate container.
- In Crohn's colitis, strictures may require using a thinner caliber colonoscope.
- Consider brush cytology or barium enema to evaluate impassable strictures.

Adapted from Itzkowitz SH, Harpaz N. Diagnosis and management of dysplasia in patients with inflammatory bowel diseases. *Gastroenterology*. 2004;126(6):1634-1648.

There are several limitations to surveillance colonoscopy and colonoscopy practices are not uniform. Multiple biopsies are needed, which is time consuming. It has been estimated that 33 biopsies are required to achieve 90% confidence to detect dysplasia if it is present.[8] There are only moderate levels of agreement among pathologists on the diagnosis of dysplasia, with better agreement for patients with high-grade dysplasia (HGD) and negative biopsies rather than low-grade dysplasia (LGD) or indefinite. Table 15-1 contains a series of recommendations based on expert opinion for the performance of surveillance colonoscopy and management of the endoscopic/histologic findings.[4]

The finding of flat HGD confirmed by two expert gastrointestinal pathologists or carcinoma in endoscopic biopsy samples is an indication for colectomy. Although somewhat controversial, there is accumulating evidence to suggest that flat LGD is also an indication for colectomy because of the relatively high rate of progression to HGD or cancer.

Dysplasia in IBD may occur in flat mucosa (endoscopically invisible) or as an elevated lesion on endoscopy. In fact, a recent study suggests that most dysplasia (89.3%) found in patients with IBD is elevated.[9-10] However some raised dysplastic lesions in IBD have endoscopic features similar to adenomas and several reports have described the conservative management of small polypoid dysplastic lesions in patients with IBD. Recent studies have demonstrated that patients with adenoma-like dysplasia-associated lesions/masses (DALMs) may be treated adequately by polypectomy and continued surveillance because of their low association with cancer, in contrast to non-adenoma-like DALMs, which still remain an indication for colectomy because of their high association with cancer.[11-15] In the absence of flat dysplasia surrounding the lesion or elsewhere in the colon, the risk of development of dysplasia or colorectal cancer was low over an 82-month follow-up period.[11,12]

Newer techniques are needed to facilitate the identification of neoplastic lesions in patients with IBD. Chromoendoscopy may be the technique most readily applicable in clinical practice.[16-18] Chromoendoscopy can improve the detection of subtle colonic lesions, raising the sensitivity of the endoscopic examination, and improve lesion characterization, increasing the specificity of the examination. Additionally, crypt architecture can be categorized using the pit pattern, aiding differentiation between neoplastic and non-neoplastic changes, and enabling the performance of targeted biopsies. Several different stains have been used including contrast stains (indigo carmine) and vital stains (methylene blue). In one study by Kiesslich, 165 patients with long-standing UC were randomized to conventional colonoscopy or colonoscopy with chromoendoscopy using 0.1% methylene blue.[19] More targeted biopsies were possible, and significantly more intraepithelial neoplasia was detected in the chromoendoscopy group (32 versus 10; $P = 0.003$). The sensitivity and specificity for differentiation between non-neoplastic and neoplastic lesions were 93%.[19] In a second back-to-back colonoscopy study, 100 patients with long-standing UC underwent conventional colonoscopy with random and directed biopsies followed by spraying with 0.1% indigo carmine and directed biopsies.[20] There was no dysplasia in 2904 nontargeted biopsies with 43 mucosal abnormalities in 20 patients in the predye spray patients, 2 of which were dysplastic. After spraying an additional 114, abnormalities were seen in 55 patients, 7 of which were dysplastic. The authors concluded that careful mucosal examination aided by pancolonic chromoendoscopy and targeted biopsies of suspicious lesions may be a more effective surveillance methodology than taking multiple nontargeted biopsies.

Given the inherent difficulties in the performance of surveillance colonoscopy, it has been suggested that chemoprevention be explored as a method to lower the risk of developing dysplasia and CRC in IBD. Chemoprevention refers to the use of drugs to reverse, suppress or to delay the process of carcinogenesis. Several agents have been suggested as chemopreventive agents including folic acid, ursodeoxycholic acid, nonsteroidal anti-inflammatory drugs (NSAIDs), and 5-aminosalicylic acids (5ASAs). A discussion of the data for and against chemoprevention is beyond the scope of this presentation, but the reader is referred to several recent reviews for additional information.[21-23] It must be made clear that there is insufficient evidence to modify present screening and surveillance practices in IBD patients on these medications and that chemoprevention is not a substitute for surveillance colonoscopy.

References

1. Eaden J. Review article: colorectal carcinoma and inflammatory bowel disease. *Aliment Pharmacol Ther.* 2004;20(Suppl 4):24-30.
2. Loftus Jr. EV, Epidemiology and risk factors for colorectal dysplasia and cancer in ulcerative colitis. *Gastroenterol Clin North Am.* 2006;35(3):517-531.
3. Friedman S, Rubin PH, Bodian C, et al. Screening and surveillance colonoscopy in chronic Crohn's colitis. *Gastroenterology.* 2001;120(4):820-826.
4. Itzkowitz SH, Harpaz N. Diagnosis and management of dysplasia in patients with inflammatory bowel diseases. *Gastroenterology.* 2004;126(6):1634-1648.
5. Itzkowitz SH, Present DH. Consensus conference: Colorectal cancer screening and surveillance in inflammatory bowel disease. *Inflamm Bowel Dis.* 2005;11(3):314-321.
6. Rutter M, Saunders B, Wilkinson K, et al. Severity of inflammation is a risk factor for colorectal neoplasia in ulcerative colitis. *Gastroenterology.* 2004;126(2):451-459.
7. Rutter MD, Saunders BP, Wilkinson KH, et al. Cancer surveillance in longstanding ulcerative colitis: endoscopic appearances help predict cancer risk. *Gut.* 2004;53(12):1813-1816.
8. Rubin CE, Haggitt RC, Burmer GC, et al. DNA aneuploidy in colonic biopsies predicts future development of dysplasia in ulcerative colitis. *Gastroenterology.* 1992;103(5):1611-1620.
9. Rutter MD, Saunders BP, Wilkinson KH, et al. Most dysplasia in ulcerative colitis is visible at colonoscopy. *Gastrointest Endosc.* 2004;60(3):334-339.
10. Itzkowitz S, Ullman T. The world isn't flat. *Gastrointest Endosc.* 2004;60(3):426-427.
11. Engelsgjerd M, Farraye FA, Odze RD. Polypectomy may be adequate treatment for adenoma-like dysplastic lesions in chronic ulcerative colitis. *Gastroenterology.* 1999;117(6):1288-1294; discussion 1488-1491.
12. Odze RD, Farraye FA, Hecht JL, Hornick JL. Long-term follow-up after polypectomy treatment for adenoma-like dysplastic lesions in ulcerative colitis. *Clin Gastroenterol Hepatol.* 2004;2(7):534-541.
13. Rubin PH, Friedman S, Harpaz N, et al. Colonoscopic polypectomy in chronic colitis: conservative management after endoscopic resection of dysplastic polyps. *Gastroenterology.* 1999;117(6):1295-1300.
14. Friedman S, Odze RD, Farraye FA. Management of neoplastic polyps in inflammatory bowel disease. *Inflamm Bowel Dis.* 2003;9(4):260-266.
15. Vieth M, Behrens H, Stolte M. Sporadic adenoma in ulcerative colitis: endoscopic resection is an adequate treatment. *Gut.* 2006;55(8):1151-1155.
16. Rutter M, Bernstein C, Matsumoto T, Kiesslich R, Neurath M. Endoscopic appearance of dysplasia in ulcerative colitis and the role of staining. *Endoscopy.* 2004;36(12):1109-1114.
17. Farraye FA, Schroy 3rd PC. Chromoendoscopy: a new vision for colonoscopic surveillance in IBD. *Gastroenterology.* 2006;131(1):323-325; discussion 325-326.
18. Thorlacius H, Toth E. Role of chromoendoscopy in colon cancer surveillance in inflammatory bowel disease. *Inflamm Bowel Dis.* 2007;13(7):911-917.
19. Kiesslich R, Fritsch J, Holtmann M, et al. Methylene blue-aided chromoendoscopy for the detection of intraepithelial neoplasia and colon cancer in ulcerative colitis. *Gastroenterology.* 2003;124(4):880-888.
20. Rutter MD, Saunders BP, Schofield G, et al. Pancolonic indigo carmine dye spraying for the detection of dysplasia in ulcerative colitis. *Gut.* 2004;53(2):256-260.
21. Croog VJ, Ullman TA, Itzkowitz SH. Chemoprevention of colorectal cancer in ulcerative colitis. *Int J Colorectal Dis.* 2003;18(5):392-400.
22. Chan EP, Lichtenstein GR. Chemoprevention: risk reduction with medical therapy of inflammatory bowel disease. *Gastroenterol Clin North Am.* 2006;35(3):675-712.
23. Levine JS, Burakoff R. Chemoprophylaxis of colorectal cancer in inflammatory bowel disease: current concepts. *Inflamm Bowel Dis.* 2007;13(10):1293-1298.

I Seem to Find Many Flat Polyps in the Cecum and Rectum of my Patients. How Should I Treat Them Other Than Sending Them to Surgery, Which Seems a Little Excessive?

Jerome D. Waye, MD

Flat polyps are problematic no matter where they are located, but especially when in the cecum. Flat polyps in the rectum are usually easily dealt with since a submucosal injection of saline is often not necessary to elevate polyps because of two reasons: 1) the rectum is below the peritoneal reflection, and deep excavations can be performed without fear of perforation, and 2) the rectum is very distensible, and also quite collapsible. The distensibility permits the rectum to act as a reservoir for stool, and the ability to contract aids in defecation. During colonoscopy, when a flat polyp is splayed out on the wall of a distended rectum, aspirating air from the rectum causes the circumference to decrease, and the footprint of the polyp decreases as well; since the polyp volume does not change, it becomes taller as the size of its base becomes smaller. This allows the endoscopist to place a snare over a polyp in the distended rectum; with air aspiration, the polyp rises up into the snare, making resection with pure coagulation current quite easy. Multiple segments can be removed in piecemeal fashion. If the polyp actually involves the dentate line, electrocautery can be painful because of cutaneous sensation. An injection of a local anesthetic can be helpful.

In the cecum, the situation is more dangerous because the distended cecal wall is relatively thin, with thickness varying from 1.7 to 2.4 mm. As in the rectum, air aspiration will result in a decreased circumference, a thicker colon wall, and a decrease in the polyp footprint. A deep excavation is not desirable with cecal polyps; therefore, for any polyp with a base greater than 1.5 cm, fluid should be injected into the submucosal space to increase the distance between the muscularis propria and the cautery resection line. Plain saline is the preferred solution, but a few drops of methylene blue can be added to color the submucosa and increase the visual contrast between the pinkish polyp lying on a blue background of injected fluid. Most endoscopists do not add epinephrine.

The amount of fluid injected is sufficient when the polyp elevates and there is a bulge in the submucosal space around the polyp base. If the benign appearing polyp does not become elevated during injection, then the injection is probably not being given in the right plane and the needle may not actually be in the submucosal space. Another reason for "nonlifting" is that the polyp is malignant and has infiltrated into the submucosa. It is imperative that the polyp itself be observed to expand and elevate with the injection, otherwise the injection has not been of benefit for polypectomy.

As long as the polyp does not involve the appendiceal orifice and go into it, most polyps in the cecum can be removed, usually in piecemeal fashion following the adequate injection of fluid into the submucosal space. Even in the cecum, after polypectomy, the base and edges can be treated with the argon plasma coagulator to ensure its complete removal.

Large sessile polyps that require special expertise in their removal are those that are greater than one-third the circumference of the bowel and cross over two haustral folds. Those that appear to be malignant (surface ulceration and/or irregularity, spontaneous bleeding) can be attempted if they elevate with a submucosal injection (tattoo) of fluid. Any polyp in a difficult location (around a fold or only seen on scope retroflexion) or that may need subsequent surgery should be marked with a permanent carbon particle submucosal injection, which will remain at the site forever.

Following piecemeal removal, several fragments need to be recovered for pathologic review. Small pieces can be suctioned into a retrieval trap, but a mesh basket is useful to collect several large fragments.

Bleeding is the major complication from removal of large sessile polyps, but immediate bleeding is usually contained at the time of polypectomy by epinephrine injection, clips,, or a thermal modality such as the argon plasma coagulator. Late bleeding may require a cathartic prep, but rarely results in the need for surgery. Perforation is unusual during piecemeal polypectomy especially if a submucosal injection was given to elevate the polyp away from the deeper tissue layers

Japanese endoscopists have pioneered the technique of endoscopic submucosal dissection, which has not been widely embraced in the Western world. This ESD procedure involves injection of a long-lasting substrate into the submucosa. After rimming the circumference of the fluid-filled bleb with a cautery-knife, the polyp is removed in one piece by cutting into the fluid-filled submucosal plane, undermining the entire polyp during its resection. The procedure is innovative as well as tedious, with a significant bleeding incidence and a 5% perforation rate, although most patients do not require surgical intervention.

References

1. Speake D, Biyani D, Frizelle FA, Watson AJ. Flat adenomas. *ANZ J Surg.* 2007;77:4-8.
2. Rembacken BJ, Fujii Tm Cairns A, Dixon MF, et al. Flat and depressed colonic neoplasms: a prospective study of 1000 colonoscopies. *UK Lancet.* 2000;355:1211-1214.
3. Hurlstone DP, Cross SS, Adam I, et al. A prospective clinicopathological and endoscopic evaluation of flat and depressed colorectal lesions in the United Kingdom. *Am J Gastroenterol.* 2003;98:2543-2549.
4. Saito Y, Uraoka T, Matsuda T, et al. Endoscopic treatment of large superficial colorectal tumors: a case series of 200 endoscopic submucosal dissections. *Gastrointest Endosc.* 2007;66:966-973.

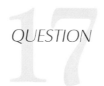

I Frequently Get Calls to Decompress a Distended Colon and the Radiologist Is Unsure if It Is a Volvulus or Pseudo-Obstruction. How Should I Approach This Technically? What Is the Role of the GI in These Conditions, and When Is a Surgical Opinion Needed?

Nirmal S. Mann, MD, MS, PhD, DSc, FRCPC, AGAF, FASGE, FACG, MACP

There are many causes of distended colon and colonic obstruction in the adult. These include toxic megacolon of inflammatory bowel disease, pseudomembranous colitis, infectious colitis, and ischemic colitis. Other causes of distended colon include benign and malignant strictures, volvulus, pseudo-obstruction, chronic constipation, fecal impaction, chronic narcotic use, and ultrashort segment Hirschsprung's disease. By definition megacolon is said to be present when on plain abdominal film the cecum or any segment of the colon is distended more than 10 cm in width.

There is no colonoscopic treatment of toxic megacolon of inflammatory bowel disease; in fact, colonoscopy is contraindicated in these cases because the risk of colonic perforation is high. These conditions should be treated with intravenous fluids, antibiotics and parenteral steroids; if there is no improvement within 24 to 48 hours, surgical intervention becomes imperative. Colonic dilation of pseudo-membranous colitis and infectious colitis should be treated with appropriate antibiotics; in rare cases, surgery may be needed. In selected cases, careful colonoscopic decompression of the unprepared colon using minimal air insufflations may be performed. Ischemic colitis may be suspected in a setting of congestive heart failure, cardiac arrhythmia, or involvement of other organs with atherosclerotic process. On plain film of the abdomen, the characteristic "thumb-printing" sign may be seen. Computerized axial tomography (CAT) scan may show abnormal thickening of the colonic wall. Colonic obstruction of acute diverticulitis should be treated with parenteral fluids and parenteral antibiotics; in acute diverticulitis, colonoscopy should not be performed.

The causes of benign colonic strictures include healed diverticulitis, endometriosis, post radiation strictures, peritoneal adhesions, and intussusception. In the management of these benign strictures, dietary modification may be needed. Endoscopic management may include balloon dilation. However, in severe cases surgical resection may be needed. Patients with extensive diverticulosis should be treated with high fiber diet, fiber supplementation and judicious use of laxatives and stool softeners. Ileocecal intussusception has a typical "coil spring" appearance on x-ray examination.

The detailed management of malignant colonic strictures is beyond the scope of this chapter. Surgery, radiotherapy, and chemotherapy have shown significant benefit; chemotherapy even in advanced metastatic disease has shown promising results. Palliation of the malignant stricture is possible by colonoscopic placement of stents.

Hirschsprung's disease is a disease of infants and children; however, ultrashort segment Hirschsprung's disease may present in adults. The diagnosis can be confirmed by motility studies, balloon test, and full-thickness biopsy of the involved segment. Treatment is usually surgical resection of the involved segment.

Acute abdominal distention commonly occurs with colonic volvulus and is present in 70% of cases. About 20% have nausea, vomiting, abdominal pain, and constipation. Colonic volvulus is the axial twisting of the colon on its vascular pedicle. In the United States, about 15% of colonic obstructions are due to volvulus; it is more common in Asia and Africa. The most common site of colonic volvulus is the sigmoid (75%), followed by cecum (20%); rare sites of colonic volvulus are splenic flexure and transverse colon. Sigmoid volvulus tends to occur more commonly in older patients, often in a setting of cardiac, renal, and pulmonary diseases; chronic constipation; laxative abuse; and mental illness. It is more common in males. Cecal volvulus is more common in women who often have a prior history of abdominal operation.

In sigmoid volvulus, the abdominal film shows markedly dilated colon and sigmoid with minimal air in the rectum. The classic radiologic feature is a distended haustral sigmoid loop. The radiologic features of cecal volvulus are dilated cecum located across the midline, distended loops of small bowel, and a single, long air-fluid level present on upright film. If there are no signs of colonic necrosis, a gentle water-soluble contrast enema may show typical bird's beak sign in sigmoid volvulus; sometimes barium enema may correct the sigmoid volvulus. In the absence of peritonitis, flexible sigmoidoscopy or colonoscopy with placement of a rectal tube may achieve colonic decompression, followed by elective sigmoid resection and coloproctostomy or end colostomy in poor surgical risk patients. Although colonoscopy has been performed successfully in patients with cecal volvulus, the thinned and ischemic cecum is prone to perforation. Operative management of cecal volvulus includes cecopexy, cecostomy, and resection. Most surgeons perform right colectomy with primary ileo-transverse colon anastomosis. In poor risk patients, colonocopic cecostomy has been performed rarely as a temporary measure to decompress the colon. The mortality rate for colonic volvulus is about 10%; however, the presence of gangrenous bowel significantly increases the mortality rate.

Acute colonic pseudo-obstruction (Ogilvie's syndrome) presents as intestinal ileus with bowel dilation and occurs in critically ill patients (eg, those with stroke, peritonitis, sepsis, myocardial infarction, and after various surgical procedures). Use of narcotics to treat post surgical pain may precipitate this condition. The patients have severe abdominal distention and no passage of stool or gas per rectum. Nausea and vomiting may be present. The abdominal distention usually is painless and there is no abdominal tenderness. The plain film of the abdomen shows dilation of the cecum and ascending colon, but sometimes the left colon is also involved. In general, "impending perforation" is diagnosed when cecal diameter exceeds 10 cm. Preventive measures included avoidance of electrolyte abnormalities, and avoidance of codeine as a narcotic. Treatment includes management of reversible underlying conditions of infection, electrolyte imbalance, dehydration, and hypotension. The patient should be NPO (not given food) and be given intravenous fluids. Check daily with abdominal films, white blood cells (WBC), and electrolytes. If perforation is suspected, prompt surgery is recommended. After 72 hours, if the cecal diameter is still > 9 cm and there are no contraindications to neostigmine, the latter is infused 1 to 2 mg over a 5-minute period. If there is no response to neostigmine, our practice is to perform a careful colonoscopy in the unprepared colon with minimal insufflation of air while vigorous suction of colonic contents is performed. It is our practice to leave a guidewire in the proximal colon as the colonoscope is withdrawn. After colonoscopy, a decompression tube is passed over the guidewire and the guidewire is withdrawn. The decompression tube is connected to slow continuous suction. If the patient's colon ejects the decompression tube, it is a good prognostic sign; it means the colonic motility is returning to normal. If the patient is not improving and is a poor surgical risk, nonsurgical cecostomy (either radiologic or endoscopic) may be performed. Surgical decompression that includes colostomy, cecostomy, or resection results in poorer outcome. The mortality rate in acute colonic pseudo-obstruction varies from 0% to 32% and is determined by comorbidity.

References

1. Ballantyne GH. Review of sigmoid volvulus: history of results of treatment. *Dis Colon Rectum*. 1982;25:494-510.
2. Grossman EM, Longo WE, Stratton MD, Virgo KS, Johnson FE. Sigmoid volvulus in Department of Veterans Affairs Medical Centers. *Dis Colon Rectum*. 2000;43:414-422.
3. Vanek VW, Al-Salti M. Acute pseudo-obstruction of the colon (Ogilvie's syndrome): An analysis of 400 cases. *Dis Colon Rectum*. 1986;29:203-207.
4. Geller A, Petersen BT, Gostout CJ. Endoscopic decompression for acute colonic pseudo-obstruction. *Gastrointest Endosc*. 1996;44:144-147.
5. Skinner M. Hirschsprung disease. *Curr Probl Surg*. 1996;32:393-405.

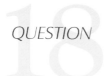

WHAT DO PEOPLE DO FOR TREATMENT OF ACHALASIA THESE DAYS? DOES IT MATTER IF THE SYMPTOMS ARE SEVERE OR IF THE PATIENT IS ELDERLY?

Terry L. Jue, MD, and Joseph Leung, MD, FRCP, FACP, FACG, FASGE

Achalasia is an esophageal motility disorder characterized by the absence of esophageal peristalsis and ineffective lower esophageal sphincter (LES) relaxation. Dysphagia to solids and liquids, heartburn, and chest pain are common symptoms. Respiratory symptoms due to aspiration can occur and progression of achalasia can lead to weight loss.

The cause of achalasia remains unknown. Acetylcholine is the neurotransmitter that causes contraction of the smooth muscle of the lower esophagus, while nitric oxide (NO) and vasoactive intestinal polypeptide (VIP) promote relaxation. In achalasia, it is believed that inflammation of the myenteric plexus of the esophagus results in loss of inhibitory signals to the lower esophagus. Unopposed stimulation of the smooth muscle causes a loss of peristalsis and failure of the LES to relax. A hypothesis suggests that a viral infection triggers inflammation of the myenteric plexus, and in genetically susceptible individuals, antibodies to the myenteric neurons of the esophagus are produced. The inflammation caused by infection and then by autoantibodies leads to a loss of inhibitory neurons resulting in achalasia.

Achalasia is uncommon, with a British study reporting an annual incidence of 1 per 100,000 individuals. Achalasia affects men and women equally, and onset can occur during any decade of life but children are seldom affected since achalasia usually does not occur before adolescence.

In a patient with achalasia, a barium swallow may show a dilated esophagus with constriction of the LES, otherwise known as a "bird's beak" appearance. Esophageal manometry will demonstrate ineffective motility of the lower esophagus and impaired LES relaxation. Although a barium study and a manometry may suggest achalasia, esophagogastroduodenoscopy (EGD) should be performed to visualize the cardia of the stomach. A tumor at the lower esophagus or at the cardia may invade the myenteric plexus, leading to secondary achalasia or "pseudoachalasia." Another less common cause of secondary achalasia is infection by *Trypanosoma cruzi*, or Chagas disease. The infection is endemic to rural, undeveloped areas of Central and South America.

Achalasia has no known cure. Treatment is palliative and focuses upon reducing LES pressure. Treatment options include medications, pneumatic balloon dilation, botulinum toxin injection of the LES, and surgical myotomy. Calcium channel blockers cause LES relaxation by inhibiting the uptake of calcium into muscle cells, while nitrates replace the depleted nitric oxide of the LES. The medications are taken 30 to 60 minutes before meals, and the improvement in dysphagia is variable. However, hypotension, headache, and peripheral edema are common unwanted effects that are not well tolerated. Tolerance to therapy occurs over time, resulting in less effect on achalasia. Hence, most patients may not respond successfully to medications alone.

Pneumatic dilation of the LES can be performed endoscopically and has a high rate of success. We recommend advancing the scope into the stomach and leaving a soft-tip guidewire across the gastroesophageal junction. Initial dilation can be performed with a 30-mm balloon inflated under fluoroscopy. At times, a "waist" is seen on the partially inflated balloon at the LES suggestive of increased muscle tone. With full balloon insufflation, this waist will resolve. The patient should be adequately sedated because balloon dilation can be uncomfortable. A good proportion of patients will have improvement in symptoms after dilation to 30 mm, but some may require repeat dilation with a 35-mm balloon. If symptoms still do not improve, dilation with a 40-mm balloon can be considered. The main risk of pneumatic dilation is esophageal perforation, which occurs at a rate of less than 3% when performed by an experienced endoscopist. The risk of perforation is highest with the first dilation. We therefore recommend performing initial dilation under fluoroscopy with a 30- or 35-mm balloon.

When injected into the lower esophagus, botulinum toxin inhibits the stimulatory effect of acetylcholine on the smooth muscle and decreases LES pressure. Botulinum toxin is commonly packaged in 100 unit (U) vials. We prefer to dilute 100 U of botulinum toxin A in 4 ml of normal saline and use a sclerotherapy needle for injection. Botulinum toxin can then be injected in a four-quadrant manner into the LES. Injections are done with 20 to 25 U into each quadrant. Doses greater than 25 U have not demonstrated greater benefit in the treatment of achalasia.

Botulinum toxin has demonstrated good results in decreasing LES tone and improving esophageal emptying. The treatment effect, however, will diminish over time and repeat injections may be necessary. Those who benefit should experience improvement of their symptoms for several months, but the duration of effect will vary for different patients, and an ideal dosing schedule has not been established. Some suggest that a treatment with 100 U of botulinum toxin initially followed by a second injection in 1 month will result in a greater durability of therapy. Contraindications to botulinum toxin include pregnancy, allergy to albumin, and reaction to prior administered botulinum toxin. Side effects can include reflux, skin rash, and chest discomfort.

Surgical myotomy for achalasia treatment involves an incision through the muscle of the LES. Myotomy has a very high rate of success in treating dysphagia, and the response usually lasts many years. When performed laparoscopically in the hands of an experienced surgeon, the procedure is well-tolerated with low rates of complication. Although surgical myotomy improves dysphagia, gastroesophageal reflux can occur after the procedure. For this reason, many surgeons will perform fundoplication at the time of myotomy. However, a comparative analysis did not find a significant improvement in postoperative reflux when fundoplication was combined with myotomy.

After a diagnosis or achalasia is made, the best approach to therapy should be decided based upon the patient's age and comorbidities. Pneumatic dilation and botulinum toxin injections have greater efficacy in patients aged 50 or older. In addition, surgical myotomy may be more difficult to perform in patients who have undergone prior dilation or botulinum toxin injections. Hence, if an achalasia patient is young and healthy, referral to an experienced surgeon for laparoscopic myotomy is the treatment of choice. In older patients with significant comorbidities, surgical myotomy may not be the best option. Pneumatic dilation has a longer effect than botulinum toxin injection, and botulinum toxin is also expensive. However, the risk of perforation, while very low, is greater with pneumatic dilation. Hence, in the patient with contraindications to surgical myotomy, life-expectancy is weighed when deciding whether to perform dilation versus botulinum toxin injection. In patients whose life-expectancy is greater than 5 years, we prefer dilation on the basis of its longer therapeutic effect. For those who presented with severe symptoms with a manometric diagnosis of vigorous achalasia, it is advisable to consider a surgical myotomy if the patient is otherwise young and healthy. If the patient is old or not a surgical candidate, botulinum toxin injection may carry a better response.

If patients begin to experience dysphagia or other manifestations of achalasia after a prior successful treatment, a repeat EGD with possible intervention should be performed. Patients should be educated that the treatment options for achalasia do not cure the disorder and that symptoms can recur. In addition, recurrence of symptoms can occur several months to years after therapy. Other health care providers should also be made aware that treatment is not curative.

References

1. Annese V, Bassotti G, Coccia G, et al. A multicentre randomized study of intrasphincteric botulinum toxin in patients with oesophageal achalasia. GISMAD Achalasia Study Group. *Gut.* 2000:46:597-600.
2. Lyass S, Thoman D, Steiner JP, et al. Current status of antireflux procedure in laparoscopic Heller myotomy. *Surg Endosc.* 2003;17:554-8.
3. Lake JM, Wong RK. Review Article: the management of achalasia—a comparison of different treatment modalities. *Aliment Pharmacol Ther.* 2006;24(6):909-18.
4. Gui D, Rossi S, Runfola M, et al. Review article: botulinum toxin in the therapy of gastrointestinal motility disorders. *Alimen Pharmacol Ther.* 2003;18(1):1-16.
5. Park W, Vaezi MF. Etiology and pathogenesis of achalasia: the current understanding. *Am J Gastroenterol.* 2005;100(6):1404-14.

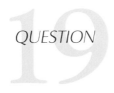

WHAT IS THE BEST BOWEL PREPARATION AND TIMING FOR AN EMERGENCY COLONOSCOPY FOR GI BLEEDING?

Jerome D. Waye, MD

Lower GI bleeding is a frightening experience, but one which often stops spontaneously. Patients who have a bloody evacuation may report that the toilet bowl is full of bright red blood, but this may not correlate with the degree or severity of bleeding, since even a small amount of blood in a toilet bowl may impart an alarming red color to the water. The two circumstances for which rectal bleeding demands colonoscopic attention is bleeding that occurs post-polypectomy, or continued bleeding that occurs spontaneously. For the most part, bleeding that occurs post-polypectomy is from a source that is known to the endoscopist and may occur anywhere up to 28 days after polypectomy. If the polypectomy was in the sigmoid colon, it is relatively easy to maneuver a scope into that area and look for a bleeding site but more difficult to reach the right colon.

Not all patients who present with rectal bleeding require emergency colonoscopy. That determination is largely based on the history of the patient. If there are 1 to 2 episodes of bleeding separated by hours or it has been several hours since the last bleeding episode, colonoscopy is usually not needed. Frequent ongoing bloody evacuations require a colonoscopic examination.

Blood is a cathartic, and a relatively good cathartic. The problem with passing the instrument retrograde through the entire colon during or just after bleeding is that clots and blood often obscure the view and cause marked darkening of the visual field, making progress difficult. The best way of handling a bleeding polypectomy site is to perform emergency endoscopy as soon as possible to see the site and stop the bleeding. Cathartics are not often needed when pursuing a post-polypectomy active bleeding site, even if located in the right colon, because the exact location is known. If the bleeding stops spontaneously, there is no benefit in prepping the bowel and looking at the polypectomy site.

Once the hemostasis cascade has resulted in cessation of hemorrhage, rebleeding from that site is uncommon.

Spontaneous bleeding on the other hand demands a clean bowel with a vigorous cathartic, a process that can often be circumvented in post-polypectomy bleeding. The colon has to be well prepared in order to find a small spontaneous bleeding source which may be an angioectasia in the right colon, or could be from a diverticulum. Fortunately, diverticular disease is the most common cause for spontaneous lower gastrointestinal hemorrhage, and most of these are located in the left colon which can be intubated relatively easily. However, even with a diverticular bleed, in order to pinpoint the source, an adequate colonoscopic preparation is mandatory. There are multiple ways of approaching the problem. Whether spontaneous bleeding or post-polypectomy hemorrhage, the best situation is for the procedure to be performed in the main endoscopy unit during daytime hours: if a cathartic is to be administered, the preparation should be timed so that the patient may be seen in the main endoscopy unit during working hours.

The best prep is a colon washout with 4 or more liters of electrolyte preparation, after which the procedure can usually be performed within 4 hours of starting the cathartic with the expectation of having a clean, but fluid filled colon. Intravenous metoclopramide (10 mg) can be given prior and every 4 hours to potentiate gastric emptying and to control nausea. In the presence of active bleeding, it is desirable to have a large fluid effluent to dilute the blood, wash the blood from the walls, and permit suction to clear the field. The electrolyte preparation can be given to the patient orally with instructions to drink the full amount of solution quickly, or can be given via a nasogastric tube. The window for emergency colonoscopy is 4 to 8 hours after beginning the preparation. There are various 2-liter electrolyte preparations on the market, but their onset of bowel activity varies from a few hours to several after ingestion and cannot be relied upon for prepping the emergency lower GI bleeder. Phospho soda and citrate of magnesia require 2 doses over a span of several hours, and the cathartic response is not reliable for emergency bleeding.

If the patient presents at 4:00 pm with postpolypectomy bleeding, emergency colonoscopy and hemostasis should be performed in the endoscopy suite. Ideally, the patient with spontaneous lower GI bleeding should be endoscoped as soon as possible, but if expertise is not available after hours it may be prudent to give support, and begin an electrolyte preparation in the early morning hours so the patient can be fully prepared to have colonoscopy performed in the main endoscopy unit at 8:00 am.

References

1. Green BT, Rockey DC, Portwood G, et al. Urgent colonoscopy for evaluation and management of acute lower gastrointestinal hemorrhage: a randomized controlled trial. *Am J Gastroenterol.* 2005;100:2395-2402.
2. Jensen DM. Management of patients with severe hematochezia—with all current evidence available. *Am J Gastroenterol.* 2005;100:2403-2406.
3. Rex DK, Lewis BS, Waye JD. Colonoscopy and endoscopic therapy for delayed post-polypectomy hemorrhage. *Gastrointest Endosc.* 1992;38:127-129.

SECTION III

ENDOSCOPIC RETROGRADE CHOLANGIOPANCREATOGRAPHY

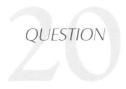

I Have a Patient With a Post-Cholecystectomy Bile Leak and Treated Him With a 7-French Stent. Four Days Later, His JP Drain Still Puts Out 300 cc/Day. What Is the Problem and What Should Be Done?

Joseph Leung, MD, FRCP, FACP, FACG, FASGE, and Simon Lo, MD, FACP

The underlying problem could be related to that fact that the stent is too small or has stent migration or associated bile duct injury.

In the investigation of postcholecystectomy (or postsurgical) bile leakage, it is important to see the leak and confirm communication between the leak and the biliary system in order to ensure that endoscopic treatment will be successful. It is important at the time of endoscopic retrograde cholangiopancreatography (ERCP) to perform an adequate cholangiogram (including, if necessary, an occlusion cholangiogram) to demonstrate the exact site of leakage (especially if clinical evidence of leakage is present). There is always controversy over whether the occlusion cholangiogram will further damage the area of the leak. However, an occlusion cholangiogram is indicated especially when leakage involves the peripheral bile ducts, such as Luschka's ducts, or if there is associated surgical trauma to the liver. Even when contrast is injected under pressure, one can stop the injection as soon as spillage of contrast is demonstrated, and further damage to the leakage area can be kept to a minimum. The concern is that if no spillage of contrast is demonstrated even on occlusion cholangiography in the presence of persistent bile leakage, it may signify a transected aberrant duct. In this case, the free transected end is leaking, whereas the communication with the biliary system is tied off. The management of this unique problem is more difficult.

A postcholecystectomy bile leak can occur at the cystic duct stump (eg, loose clip or failure to clip or ligate the cystic duct), from damaged aberrant Luschka's ducts, from damage to the common bile duct, or less commonly, transaction of aberrant ducts. Although the literature suggest that simple bile leak usually closes after a few days if adequate internal drainage is provided, it may take up to 1 week before the leak resolves completely. It is important to monitor the amount of drainage from the Jackson-Pratt (JP) drain; a decreasing trend is expected with adequate drainage.

Bile tends to flow in the path of least resistance. In the normal steady state, the resting sphincter pressure maintains a positive hydrostatic pressure within the biliary system. In the presence of a bile leak or bile duct injury, bile will flow through the vent and collect around the subhepatic space.

The usual recommendation for managing a bile leak is a biliary papillotomy either with or without placement of an indwelling biliary stent. More recent studies showed that placement of a large biliary stent (preferably a 10-French (Fr) [2.8 mm internal] diameter straight stent) is sufficient to control simple bile leaks from the cystic duct stump or aberrant Luschka's ducts, and papillotomy for single stent placement is not necessary. Depending on the size of the leak (diameter of cystic duct) and location of the stent, placement of a 7-Fr stent (1.8 mm internal diameter) may not be sufficient to divert the bile from the site of leakage if the leak is considerably larger than the lumen of the stent. Persistence of bile leakage has been reported in this situation, and it may be necessary to insert multiple stents to overcome a large bile leak.

The presence of an obstructing factor, including a retained stone, may also impede the flow of bile and cause persistent bile leakage. In this situation, a papillotomy is required to remove the common bile duct (CBD) stone and then placement of a 10-Fr stent to control bile leakage.

In less common situations, there may be cautery or clip injury to the bile duct, resulting in bile duct stenosis (or stricture) that perpetuates the leak. In such cases, prolonged stenting with an indwelling larger stent may be necessary.

Lastly, the stent could have migrated up the bile duct (especially if a prior papillotomy was performed) and, therefore, drainage affected. Alternatively, the stent could have migrated out of the bile duct, thus not providing any effective drainage. This can be checked and ruled out easily by taking a plain x-ray of the abdomen to determine the location of the stent.

My personal approach to management of an uncomplicated bile leak from the cystic duct stump or aberrant Luschka's ducts is placement of a 10-Fr stent. This provides much better drainage than a 7-Fr stent. It is not necessary to perform a biliary papillotomy (unless there is difficulty with access and deep cannulation) although papillotomy alone has been reported to be effective in treating a bile leak. Usually, I prefer to place the proximal end of the stent above the insertion of the cystic duct to ensure bile flowing down is collected by the stent. Sometimes, the stent can migrate, and one thing I can do is to shape the stent to create a curvature and to open the proximal and distal flaps to minimize the risk of stent migration.

The management will be very different if I cannot demonstrate any contrast spillage upon cholangiogram. This may be a result of tying off an aberrant duct with a free leakage from the transected end. We should maintain a high index of suspicion if we cannot demonstrate a leak in the presence of clinical bile leakage. It is useful to count the number of intrahepatic ductal segments and determine if there is an obvious absence of intrahepatic ducts. An EHIDA scan can be performed to document the leak, and a magnetic resonance cholangiogram may demonstrate the "absent" intrahepatic ducts not seen on endoscopic retrograde cholangiography. If this is confirmed, we may need to consult interventional radiology to access the isolated system and determine if internal connectivity can be achieved. In most situations, surgical drainage and a bilioenteric anastomosis may be necessary to control the bile leakage.

In the presence of documented bile leakage, it is important to drain the subhepatic collection of bile even when internal drainage with an indwelling stent is successful in order to avoid infection and abscess formation.

Is There a Role for Metal Stents in Benign Bile Duct Strictures? When Should I Use Plastic Stents in This Setting?

Joseph Leung, MD, FRCP, FACP, FACG, FASGE

The short answer to the first question is *no*. We do not have the right metal stents at this point, although self-expandable metal stents (SEMS) have been tried on patients with refractory strictures. Stents with a different design are available outside of the United States (US) market and may offer an advantage over the currently available metal stents in the US.

Two factors need to be considered in the management of benign bile duct stricture: 1) what is the presumed cause of the benign stricture, and 2) is it likely to respond to treatment within the planned interval of endoscopic therapy. Considering all of the morbidity involved with repeat stent exchange, when should one declare a failure of stenting with plastic stents and then consider surgical revision or if metal stent(s) should be tried as an alternative treatment?

Benign bile duct strictures often complicate surgery secondary to traumatic or ischemic injury following laparoscopic cholecystectomy and less commonly as a result of a direct anastomosis or a bilio-enteric anastomosis. The involvement of the bifurcation with or without prior surgical anastomosis poses a challenge to endoscopic therapy. Other benign causes of bile duct obstruction are chronic pancreatitis involving the retropancreatic portion of the distal bile duct and anastomotic stricture following liver transplantation.

The mainstay treatment for nonoperative management of benign bile duct stricture has been endoscopic stenting with single or multiple large bore plastic stents and regular stent change to minimize the risk of blockage and cholangitis. For tight ischemic strictures, balloon dilation is often necessary prior to stent placement (Figure 21-1). A word of

Figure 21-1. (A) Benign common bile duct (CBD) stricture following liver transplantation. (B) Balloon dilation of CBD stricture.

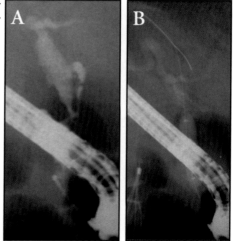

Figure 21-2. (A) Benign postoperative bile duct stricture. (B) Two stents inserted across benign bile duct stricture.

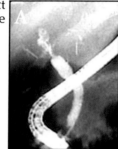 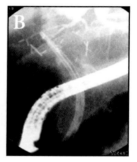

caution is overly aggressive dilation may lead to perforation because of the tight fibrous stricture, and an oversized balloon can damage the normal bile duct above or below the stricture. Balloon dilation is usually not advisable in the immediate postoperative period, especially in post-transplant strictures.

Multiple stent placement is not common, especially in the community setting, because of the difficulty in recannulation and negotiating the stricture. However, the literature suggests the use of multiple plastic stents can help to dilate and maintain patency of the stricture (Figure 21-2). It is usually recommended that a biliary papillotomy be performed to accommodate two or more stents to minimize the risk of poststenting pancreatitis. However, this does not seem to be a significant problem when an increasing number of stents was placed over an extended period. A prior biliary papillotomy certainly facilitates repeat cannulation and negotiation with a guidewire. The newly introduced Fusion OASIS system (Cook Endoscopy, Winston-Salem, NC) with the ability for intraductal release (IDR) of the guidewire has revolutionized the practice of multiple stent placement. The ability to release the guidewire within the bile duct after the first stent deployment allows the guidewire to stay across the stricture and facilitates placement of subsequent stents without having to recannulate or renegotiate the stricture (Figure 21-3). In vitro testing with an endoscopic retrograde cholangiopancreatography (ERCP) simulator showed that there is a significant reduction in the total time taken to deploy three stents

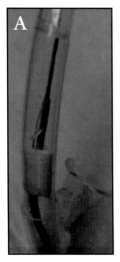
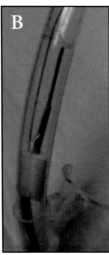

Figure 21-3. (A) Animation showing guidewire inserted through side port of inner catheter and stent "trapped" between the guidewire and inner catheter. Stent cannot be deployed until the guidewire is freed. (B) IDR of guidewire and proximal tip of guidewire is alongside the stent across the stricture in the artificial bile duct. The stent can now be deployed by pulling back on the inner catheter. Since guidewire is across stricture, a second stent can be inserted without having to recannulate or renegotiate the stricture.

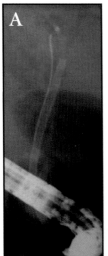
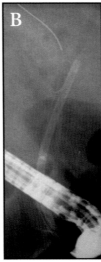
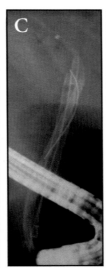

Figure 21-4. (A,B) Radiograph showing single stent deployment after IDR. (C) Radiograph showing that triple stents can be deployed across a benign bile duct stricture while maintaining the guidewire through the bile duct obstruction.

using the Fusion system (Figure 21-4) compared to another form of short wire technology, which requires recannulation of the bile duct and stricture.

The aim of stenting today is to place as many stents as possible (limited by the size of the normal portion of the bile duct) to keep the stricture open.[1,2] Stents are usually left in for 3 months with repeat dilation and stent exchange for up to 1 year. After that, the stents are removed and the patient observed for evidence of stricture recurrence. Because the distal tip of the stent is often left in the duodenum (for ease of subsequent exchange), this predisposes the patient to duodenal biliary reflux and contamination of the biliary system. One major problem I encountered with prolonged stenting is sludge/stone formation above the stricture that requires clearance prior to stent replacement. Prophylactic antibiotic therapy does not seem to prevent this complication.

Strictures complicating ischemic changes without direct duct injury are more likely to respond to endoscopic stenting. On the other hand, clip injury to the bile duct, be it partial or complete, poses a technical challenge to the management because of the difficulty of opening the clip. Aberrant duct injury is difficult to treat with the endoscopic approach because of limited or no access distally, and these cases may need surgical correction or interventional radiology. Strictures involving the bifurcation are more difficult to manage because of multiple segment involvement. Although multiple stents can be placed into each subsegment, as described by Costamagna et al,[1] it is technically challenging.

Strictures complicating chronic pancreatitis do not respond well to endoscopic stenting despite the use of multiple stents because of the inflammation and calcified pancreatic tissue in the head of the pancreas. Overall, the results with plastic stent treatment of benign stricture associated with chronic pancreatitis have been rather disappointing. In early reports, open mesh metal expandable stents have been used in some of these patients. However, because of the risk of tissue in-growth and subsequent blockage of the metal stents in a benign condition, this has never evolved into a common practice.

Potential benefits may come from the newly introduced fully covered metal stents, which are claimed to be removable. If this is true, it will certainly facilitate the management of patients with refractory benign bile duct stricture because these stents can expand to a much larger internal diameter and provide support for the stricture and drainage. The larger lumen may offer a prolonged patency and minimizes the morbidity of repeat stent exchange. The stent that can be removed would allow us to evaluate the effect of prolonged stenting. However, covered metal stents are more prone to migration. The currently available covered wall stents still have bare wires at the proximal and distal end, and stent migration can potentially bury the wires into the tissue, making subsequent removal more risky. Until a stent with a well-designed removal mechanism is available, the true benefits of metal stents in benign bile duct obstruction remain speculative.

Post-transplant bile duct strictures may be more difficult to manage due to the anastomotic nature of the cholechocholedochotomy. Balloon dilation is certainly not recommended in the early postoperative period. I prefer to place a single 10-French stent across the stricture to provide initial drainage and to consider balloon dilation after 3 months of stenting. It has been suggested that immunosuppressive agents used in the patient may contribute to sludge formation. As a result, I have observed early occurrence of sludge and intrahepatic stone formation above the stricture, and these patients may require stent exchange sooner than the suggested 3-month interval. Long-term improvement following dilation and stenting is also less satisfactory compared to postcholecystectomy strictures. In refractory cases, I have attempted to use covered expandable metal stents to manage the bile duct obstruction in place of surgical revision. However, my early experience has not been encouraging due to the migration of the covered stents.

References

1. Costamagna G, Pandolfi M, Mutignani M, Spada C, Perri V. Long-term results of endoscopic management of postoperative bile duct strictures with increasing number of stents. *Gastrointest Endosc.* 2001;54:162-168.
2. Bergman J, Burgemeister L, Bruno M, et al. Long-term follow up after biliary stent placement for postoperative bile duct stenosis. *Gastrointest Endosc.* 2001;54:154-161.

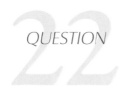
WHY IS BALLOON SPHINCTEROPLASTY STILL BEING PRACTICED, AND WHEN SHOULD WE CONSIDER THIS TREATMENT OPTION?

Rajesh Gupta, MD, DM, and D. Nageshwar Reddy, MD, DM, FRCP, DSc

Endoscopic balloon sphincteroplasty (EBS) was proposed as an alternative to endoscopic sphincterotomy (ES) in 1983.[1] The proponents of EBS believe that it preserves the function of sphincter of oddi and decreases the potential risk of bacterial contamination of the biliary tree. This in turn decreases the risk of short- and long-term complications. The subanalysis of the studies have shown that the most significant effect of EBS on short- and long-term complications was on lowering the risk of cholecystitis, and this influenced the overall risk of infections. This is an important issue in patients with an intact gallbladder, especially those who do not undergo cholecystectomy. In regards to long-term complications, there is a significantly decreased risk in patients undergoing EBS. It is this decreased risk of long-term complications that most proponents of EBS emphasize.

Several studies have shown that EBS has lower rates of bleeding and perforation as compared to ES. A recent meta-analysis has reported 0.1% overall risk of bleeding with EBS as compared to 4.8% with ES. It has been shown to be safe even in patients with coagulopathy who otherwise carry a 6% to 14% mortality with ES.[2,3] Similarly, the risk of perforation was reported to be lower with EBS as compared to ES (0% to 1% versus 1% to 2%). Since EBS carries a lower rate of bleeding, it is a safer alternative to ES not only in patients with coagulopathy but with difficult anatomy, such as those with Billroth II procedure or Roux-en-y procedures and duodenal diverticulum. Two studies involving patients with Billroth II procedures reported no bleeding complications with EBS.

Most endoscopists do not use EBS due to the fear of increased risk of pancreatitis.[4] Several randomized controlled trials have demonstrated higher rates of pancreatitis with EBS in comparison to ES (8.6% versus 4.3%). It is interesting to note that the risk of pancreatitis with EBS was more in western trials than Asian trials. The possible explanation could be the age difference of patients in these two groups. The Western trials included mainly younger patients (<60 years), while Asian trials were composed of elderly patients (mean age 60 years). However, it is neither reasonable nor justifiable to abandon EBS altogether due to fear of pancreatitis.

There is little doubt that ES is superior to EBS in overall stone extraction (95% versus 90%). EBS creates a smaller passage for clearance of bile duct stones in comparison to ES, and because of this, patients undergoing EBS require significantly more often mechanical lithotripsy for common bile duct (CBD) stone clearance than those who undergo ES. In our institute, we apply a combined technique of EBS with a 15-mm controlled radial expansion (CRE) balloon in select patients with small papilla or difficult ampullary anatomy for clearance of a large CBD stone. By this technique, we have achieved better CBD stone extraction rates without increasing the risk of complications. No data are available regarding the impact of ES and EBS on cost of the procedure, quality of life scores, or length of hospital stay. There is no significant difference in short-term mortality due to complications in ES or EBS.

EBS has a definite role in certain clinical situations. It is safer than ES in patients with coagulopathy and difficult ampullary anatomy. It is not justified to abandon this procedure altogether due to fear of pancreatitis.

References

1. Staritz M, Eve E, Myer zum Buschenfelde KH. Endoscopic papillary dilation (EPD) for the treatment of common bile duct stones and papillary stenosis. *Endoscopy.* 1983;15:117-118.
2. Baron T, Harewood C. Endoscopic balloon dilatation of the biliary sphincter compared to endoscopic biliary sphincterotomy for removal of common bile duct stones during ERCP, metanalysis of randomized controlled trials. *Am J Gastro Entrol.* 2004;99:1455-1460.
3. Weinberg BM, Shindy W, Lo S. Endoscopic balloon sphincter dilation (sphincteroplasty) versus sphincterotomy for common bile duct stones. *Cochrane Database of Systemic Reviews.* 2006;4:Art No. CD004890.
4. Di Sario JA, Freeman ML, Bjorkman DT, et al. Endoscopic balloon dilatation compared with sphincterotomy for extraction of bile duct stones: preliminary results. *Gastroenterology.* 2004;127:1291-1299.

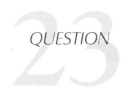

HOW DO WE MANAGE A PATIENT WITH A 10-CM PSEUDOCYST WHO IS CURRENTLY ASYMPTOMATIC?

Richard A. Kozarek, MD

Pseudocyst size is less important than the clinical context of the patient. How certain are you that the cystic lesion noted on computed tomography (CT) scan or ultrasound (US) imaging is actually a pseudocyst? For instance, a middle-aged female patient with vague abdominal symptoms who is found to have a cystic mass of any size with abdominal imaging is much more likely to have a cystic neoplasm if there has been no antecedent history of pancreatitis. Likewise, patients with intraductal papillary mucin-producing neoplasm (IPMN) or mucinous cystadenoma of the pancreas, a premalignant condition, can occasionally present with obstructive pancreatitis. The presence of a cystic lesion at the onset of pancreatitis is crucial to distinguishing a neoplastic condition from a true pseudocyst, which is the consequence of a ductal disruption and the body's containment of that disruption by a wall of inflammatory and fibrous tissue.

Pseudocysts that occur in the setting of chronic pancreatitis usually are the consequences of increased duct pressure with or without superimposed acute parenchymal inflammation.[1] There is often a stone or a stricture downstream from the site of ductal disruption. If walled off, a pseudocyst occurs. Leaks that are not walled off may be associated with high amylase pleural effusions, pancreatic ascites, or fistulization into contiguous organs. As a result of a fixed ductal obstruction, pseudocysts that occur in a patient with chronic pancreatitis are less likely to resolve spontaneously (Figures 23-1 and 23-2).

Most pancreatic fluid collections that occur in the setting of acute pancreatitis are not pseudocysts, and over three-quarters resolve over 4 to 6 weeks. Most pancreatic necrosis is not a pseudocyst, although it too is associated with a ductal leak in most patients. Necrosis frequently results in a collection of debris-filled pancreatic juice that is

Figure 23-1. Abdominal CT demonstrates a 10-cm pseudocyst (arrow) in an asymptomatic patient with hereditary pancreatitis. The patient had previous cystgastrostomy 20 years prior.

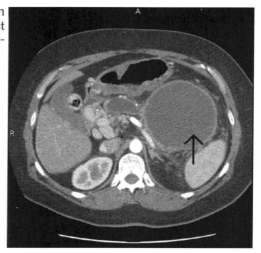

Figure 23-2. Endoscopic compression by pseudocyst in the patient depicted in Figure 23-1. As the patient had splenic and portal vein thromboses with varices, she was initially followed conservatively elsewhere.

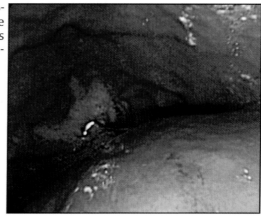

anatomically constrained by the lesser sac. CT scanning notoriously overestimates the liquid component of the collection, and US or endoscopic ultrasound (EUS) may be required to distinguish this from a pseudocyst. Other clues include the irregularity and variable thickness of the wall, nonenhancement of the pancreatic parenchyma on the early arterial phase of a pancreatic protocol CT, and the stormy clinical course of the patient to include multisystem organ failure (MSOF) and bacterial translocation from the gut with superinfection of the necrotic tissue and fluid. Pseudocysts may be a consequence of evolving pancreatic necrosis, but this often occurs several months after a severe attack of pancreatitis and occurs when the majority of necrotic tissue has liquefied and a true fibrous "rind" has formed around the fluid collection.

Pseudocysts that occur in the setting of acute pancreatitis are usually spherical, take 6 to 8 weeks to "mature," and historically were felt to be associated with a high complication rate if not treated. This was at a time that treatment consisted primarily of surgical cystgastrostomy or Roux-en-y cystojejunostomy. The maxim was that pseudocysts 6 cm or larger present for more than 6 weeks required drainage. It was in that background that percutaneous drainage of pseudocysts was popularized in an attempt to obviate surgery. Subsequently, endoscopic drainage was described as a means to avoid an indwelling percutaneous catheter.[1] The latter resulted in a long-term pancreatic fistula in 10% to 20% of patients, most of whom had a downstream ductal obstruction or the disconnected pancreatic duct syndrome.

Seminal work from the University of Minnesota randomizing asymptomatic patients with acute pseudocysts to surgery or expectant follow-up changed my treatment paradigm over 15 years ago. These investigators found a relatively low risk of pseudocyst complications as long as the diameter of the pseudocyst was stable or decreasing in size. Additional studies suggest that the 7% to 25% complication rates published in patients with pseudocyst occurred early in the clinical course or in the setting of enlarging fluid collections, most of which were symptomatic. These complications can include bleeding with pseudoaneurysm formation, obstruction of contiguous organs (bile duct, cholestasis/jaundice; stomach/duodenum, gastric outlet obstruction), cyst infection, and occasional cyst leak with free rupture but more commonly fistulization into contiguous organs.

What has changed in the last decade that allows us to follow a patient with a 10-cm pancreatic fluid collection and not recommend intervention? Imaging has improved dramatically, and CT scans, secretin magnetic resonance cholangiopancreatography (MRCP) scans,[2] and EUS with or without sampling of the cyst fluid have improved our ability to distinguish cystic neoplasms from pseudocysts, thereby eliminating patients with potential neoplasms early in the course.[3,4] We have a better understanding of acute pancreatic fluid collections because serial CT scans have demonstrated that most collections associated with acute pancreatitis resolve. Moreover, as noted previously, the majority of patients with an enlarging collection or complication of pseudocyst are not asymptomatic. Finally, we now recognize that evolving pancreatic necrosis is not a pseudocyst and that the morbidity and mortality associated with this condition are at least a log factor higher than in the setting of an acute or chronic pancreatic pseudocyst.[1]

So, if I am sure that this 10-cm fluid collection is a pseudocyst, that the patient is eating and asymptomatic, and that the cyst is stable or slowly being reabsorbed, why not follow it? How often the patient needs to be scanned, sounded, or palpated is contingent upon whether the patient is recovering from acute pancreatitis or the cyst was found incidentally in a patient with chronic pancreatitis. In the former setting, repeat imaging every 4 to 6 weeks seems reasonable, eventually increasing imaging intervals to every 5 to 6 months. In patients with chronic pancreatitis, in turn, a repeat CT or ultrasound should be considered at 1 month, and repeated at 3 and 9 to 12 months if the patient remains asymptomatic. Alternatively, because pseudocysts that occur in patients with chronic pancreatitis usually have a downstream stone or stricture preventing ultimate pseudocyst resolution, this latter situation is considered by some practitioners to be an absolute indication for intervention, regardless of the presence of symptoms.

References

1. Kozarek RA, Traverso LW. Pancreatic fistulas: etiology, consequences, and treatment. Review. *Gastroenterologist*. 1996;4:238-244.
2. Arvanitakis M, Delhaye M, De Maertelaere V, et al. Computed tomography and magnetic resonance imaging in the assessment of acute pancreatitis. *Gastroenterology*. 2004;126:715-723.
3. Singhal D, Kakodkar R, Sud R, Chaudhary A. Issues in management of pancreatic pseudocysts: review. *JOP*. 2006;7:502-507.
4. Brugge WR, Lauwers GY, Sahani D, et al. Cystic neoplasms of the pancreas: review. *N Engl J Med*. 2004;351:1218-1226.

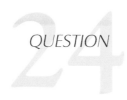
WHAT IF THE PANCREATIC CYST HAS PERSISTED FOR MORE THAN 1 YEAR AND IS NOT RESOLVING?

Richard A. Kozarek, MD

Nonresolving "pseudocysts" occur in three separate situations. The first is in the setting of a misdiagnosis; the second occurs in slowly resolving/liquefying pancreatic necrosis, which is often associated with a disconnected pancreatic duct downstream. The third is perhaps most common and occurs when there is a downstream stricture or stone in the setting of chronic pancreatitis.[1]

The vast majority of pseudocysts can be distinguished from cystic neoplasms of the pancreas by clinical history. A cystic pancreatic mass without antecedent pancreatitis is neoplastic until proven otherwise. Likewise, a patient who already has a cyst during his or her index episode of pancreatitis should be considered to have a cystic neoplasm. Clinically, mucinous cystic neoplasms of the pancreas are considered premalignant. Whereas mucinous cystadenomas frequently occur in younger or middle-aged women and have no communication with the pancreatic duct, intraductal papillary mucinous neoplasms (IPMN) are more common in elderly men, can be multifocal, and originate in side branches or the main pancreatic duct. The latter have a 50% malignant potential and a higher incidence of cysts being mistaken for pseudocysts. From an imaging perspective, cystic neoplasms are often thick walled, multilocular, have significant septae or solid components, and IPMN will frequently show a ductal communication with secretin—magnetic resonance cholangiopancreatography (MRCP) or endoscopic retrograde cholangiopancreatography (ERCP) studies. Direct pancreatoscopy and intraductal ultrasound (IDUS) are also being increasingly utilized for diagnosis and staging. If computed tomography (CT) or magnetic resonance imaging (MRI)/MRCP evaluations remain nondiagnostic, most clinicians feel that cyst analysis, either by percutaneous or endoscopic

Table 24-1

Analysis of Cyst Fluid

	Viscosity	Amylase	CEA	Cytology
Pseudocyst	Low	High	Low	-
IPMN	High	High	High	+/-
MCA	High	Low	High	+/-
SCA	Low	Low	Low	-

IPMN = intraductal papillary mucinous neoplasm
MCA = mucinous cystadenoma/adenocarcinoma
SCA = serous cystadenoma

ultrasound (EUS) aspirate, is essential. Mucinous cystadenomas/adenocarcinomas and IPMNs have high fluid viscosity (string sign) and often have high cyst carcinoembryonic antigen (CEA) levels and variable cytology results. Pseudocysts and IPMN lesions have high amylase levels in the aspirate. Table 24-1 summarizes cyst fluid analysis in various cystic lesions of the pancreas, to include serous cystadenomas, a condition generally not considered premalignant.

Pancreatic necrosis is commonly misdiagnosed as pseudocyst, particularly in the sub-acute phase. As noted in the previous question, CT scans notoriously overestimate the fluid component of the collection. Abdominal ultrasound or EUS may prove beneficial, but irregular rind and shape of the fluid collection and clinical course of the patient are often more helpful.[2] Attempting to treat these collections surgically, percutaneously, or endoscopically may be associated with iatrogenic infection when the fluid component is drained and residual necrosis is exposed to enteric flora. It is not unusual that necrotic debris can fill the lesser sac for a year or more after severe pancreatic necrosis, particularly if there is a disconnected pancreatic duct tail leaking into the collection.[3,4]

Finally, persistent pseudocysts are often associated with pancreatic duct strictures or stones in patients with chronic pancreatitis. Two-thirds of these patients are noted to have a downstream leak that perpetuates the pseudocyst.

As an example, the cyst has been present for 1 year. Percutaneous aspiration demonstrated high amylase and a negative cytology. One week later, the patient developed fever, chills, and abdominal pain. Abdominal CT demonstrated no change in the 10-cm pseudocyst (Figure 24-1). How do we treat this patient now? How do we approach a patient such as this, even if asymptomatic?

When deemed appropriate, pancreatic pseudocysts can be drained surgically (cystgastrostomy, Roux-en-y cystojejunostomy, external drainage), percutaneously, or endoscopically. In my institution, such patients are evaluated by a multidisciplinary team consisting of an interventional radiologist, pancreaticobiliary surgeon, and therapeutic endoscopist.[1] In many places, however, I predict that the treatment plan is contingent upon local expertise or which specialist touches the patient first. From my perspective, I believe that "pseudocysts" with considerable

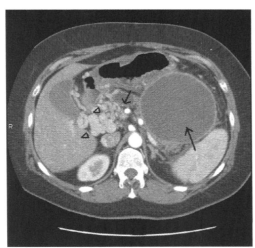

Figure 24-1. Arrows demonstrate large and small pseudocysts in the patient depicted in Question 23. Arrowheads outline large periportal varices in the setting of portal vein thrombosis. Symptoms included pain, nausea/vomiting, and fever to 39.5°C.

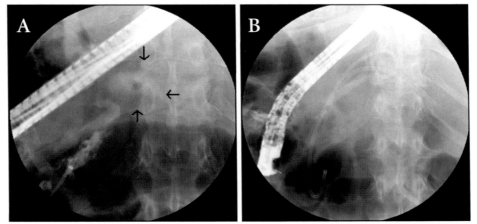

Figure 24-2. (A) Pancreatogram demonstrates severe chronic pancreatitis with pseudocyst in proximal body (B) treated with straight and pigtail transpapillary stents.

necrotic debris are better handled surgically or by placement of multiple, large caliber percutaneous drains. Likewise, patients who do not have a contiguous stomach or bowel loop to fistulize through to gain access into the cyst cavity are better handled nonendoscopically. Most pseudocysts, however, are fair game for endoscopists.

Although small pseudocysts spontaneously resolve following transpapillary stenting of a ductal disruption, this patient with a 10-cm lesion would be handled better with a "belt and suspenders" approach. The latter would include obtaining a pancreatogram, treatment of any downstream stricture or stone, and bridging the ductal disruption, if seen and technically possible, with a transpapillary stent (Figure 24-2). It would also include treating the consequence of the ductal disruption by transgastric or transduodenal pseudocyst entry followed by placement of an indwelling stent.[5] Although the techniques have been refined since my initial description of pseudocyst drainage over 2 decades ago (Figure 24-3) (fistulotome versus Seldinger needle access into the cavity, balloon dilation of the tract, EUS localization versus contrast injection into the pseudocyst), studies

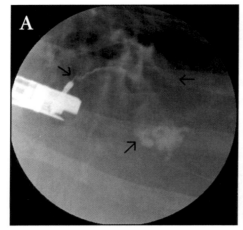

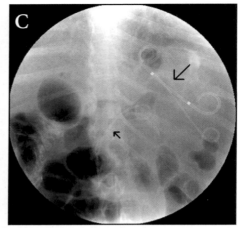

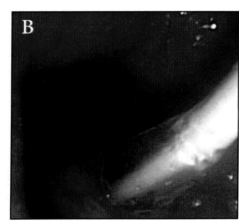

Figure 24-3. (A) Following transgastric puncture and contrast injection (arrows, (B) and balloon dilation of the tract, (C) 2 transgastric stents were placed into the pseudocyst (large arrow). Note trans-papillary stents into the smaller pseudocyst (small arrow).

suggest comparable results for endoscopy as compared with surgery or percutaneous drainage in properly selected patients. Thus, 80% to 90% of patients can be technically drained, complication rates approximate 10% to 15% contingent upon methodology, and recurrence rates approach 5% to 15%; this is in part a consequence of the disconnected duct syndrome or downstream pancreatic duct strictures or stones. EUS drainage has not been definitively shown to increase the safety or improve outcomes compared to endo-scopic drainage alone.[2] It does make sense, however, to consider EUS localization if there is no pseudocyst bulge on the stomach or duodenum or if there is splenic/portal vein thrombosis and concern about incising into a perigastric/enteric varix.

In the case depicted in Figures 24-1 to 24-4, adequate treatment required approaching an obstructed duct as well as the collection itself. Fortunately, this patient, who grew out streptococcus from her 10-cm pseudocyst, did well clinically, had all stents retrieved after 4 weeks, and has not experienced a recurrence at 12 months (Figure 24-4).

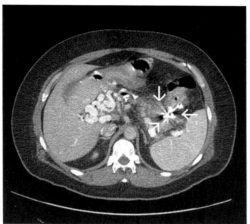

Figure 24-4. Arrows demonstrate stents in decompressed pseudocyst. The patient became asymptomatic in 24 hours and had stents retrieved at 4 weeks.

References

1. Kozarek R. Pancreatic duct leaks and pseudocysts. In: Ginsberg G, Kochman M, Norton I, Gastout C, eds. *Clinical Gastrointestinal Endoscopy*. Philadelphia, PA: WB Saunders Co; 2005:807-820.
2. Kahaleh M, Shami VM, Conaway MR, et al. Endoscopic ultrasound drainage of pancreatic pseudocyst: a prospective comparison with conventional endoscopic drainage. *Endoscopy*. 2006;38:355-359.
3. Fotoohi M, Traverso LW. Pancreatic necrosis: paradigm of a multidisciplinary team: review. *Adv Surg*. 2006;40:107-118.
4. Papachristou GI, Takahashi N, Chahal P, Sarr MG, Baron TH. Peroral endoscopic drainage/debridement of walled-off pancreatic necrosis. *Ann Surg*. 2007;245:943-951.
5. Hookey LC, Debroux S, Delhaye M, et al. Endoscopic drainage of pancreatic-fluid collections in 116 patients: a comparison of etiologies, drainage techniques, and outcomes. *Gastrointest Endosc*. 2006;63:635-643.

What Is the Best Endoscopic Method to Diagnose Pancreatic Cancer? What Is the Best Way to Sample Tissue to Diagnose Suspected Bile Duct Cancer?

John G. Lee, MD

The diagnosis of pancreatic cancer requires histological or cytological confirmation in the United States because most physicians and patients will only accept a definitive diagnosis, whereas in Japan, for example, most cancers are diagnosed on clinical and radiological findings alone. In addition, a definitive diagnosis is required to initiate treatment since oncologists will not treat based on a clinical diagnosis (sometimes even in patients with radiographical evidence of metastasis) or on elevated CA 19-9 level, however compelling it may be. Many surgeons also request a definitive diagnosis before operating because pancreatic resection has significant morbidity and smaller but a very real mortality rate associated with it even in the very "best" centers. We now know that chronic pancreatitis and autoimmune pancreatitis can present virtually identical to pancreatic cancer yet require very different therapies. Therefore, endoscopic diagnosis of pancreatic cancer requires either biopsy or cytology.

Endoscopic forceps biopsy is possible when pancreatic cancer invades into the bowel; however, apparent duodenal mucosal invasion often just represents inflammatory reaction, decreasing its positive predictive value well below 100%. Endoscopic biopsy can also be done via the bile duct in patients with biliary obstruction and/or via the pancreatic duct, especially in patients with intraductal papillary mucinous neoplasms (IPMN) who have a grossly dilated pancreatic duct (Figure 25-1). These methods are useless in patients with small tumors (ie, the patient with the highest chance of being cured). My feeling is that endoscopic intraductal biopsies are not practical or feasible in routine clinical practice because of the technical difficulty and low tissue yield. Directed biopsies using a pancreatoscope should increase the yield but are even more cumbersome, time consuming, and

Figure 25-1. "Blind" endoscopic biopsy of a cholangiocarcinoma using regular biopsy forceps.

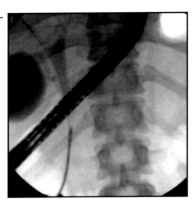

not widely available. Thus, the best and only endoscopic method for obtaining histological diagnosis of pancreatic cancer in most cases is to perform forceps biopsy of tumor invading into the gastric or duodenal wall. The prevalence of such invasion is unknown but is fairly uncommon in my clinical experience.

Brush cytology from biliary and/or pancreatic stricture can yield a positive cytologic diagnosis in about one-third of cases.[1] The yield in routine clinical practice is probably lower since results reported in published studies from experienced centers represent the very best case scenarios. Still, this is the only method available in many units and thus by default represents the best and only method of diagnosing pancreatic cancer endoscopically.

The most accurate endoscopic method to diagnose pancreatic cancer is by endoscopic ultrasound (EUS) and fine needle aspiration (FNA).[2] EUS can easily detect lesions in the 3 to 4 mm range, which is far better than computed tomography (CT), magnetic resonance imaging (MRI), or any other imaging modality and is more accurate than surgical exploration. EUS FNA is easily possible in such small lesions and can be used to obtain a definitive cytologic diagnosis with sensitivity >90%. In our experience, about half of the patients with even large tumor in EUS present with either a negative or equivocal CT scan. A normal EUS has an essentially perfect negative predictive value, meaning that a normal EUS rules out pancreatic cancer.[3] EUS is the only method that can be used to detect and mark very small lesions (usually <1 cm).[4] Our approach is to tattoo this small lesion at the time of EUS to facilitate laparoscopic wedge or partial resection (Figure 25-2). EUS FNA is also far safer than endoscopic retrograde cholangiopancreatography (ERCP) with a complication rate of around 0.1% to 0.5% and can also be used to accurately stage the disease. On the other hand, EUS FNA equipment is not always available, and technical expertise is even more limited in the United States.

Should you do ERCP and/or EUS? I think the most logical approach is to start with EUS FNA (the only endoscopic method that can diagnose a tumor without invasion into the bile or pancreatic duct) followed by ERCP and stenting only in patients with obstructive jaundice.

In conclusion, the best endoscopic method to diagnose pancreatic cancer is EUS FNA. In addition, the very high negative predictive value of a normal EUS makes it the only modality that I would feel comfortable in using to exclude the possibility of cancer. If unavailable, the patient with suspected pancreatic cancer should be

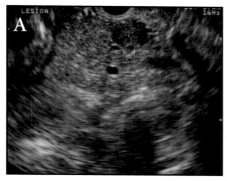

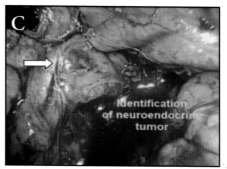

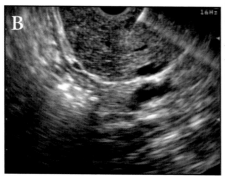

Figure 25-2. (A) EUS shows a 7-mm neuroendocrine tumor in the pancreas. (B) EUS-guided tattoo of the tumor using India ink is performed to facilitate intraoperative visualization. Note the hyperechoic blush from the injection. (C) Laparoscopic visualization of the neuroendocrine tumor with India ink tattoo.

referred to a center with EUS FNA. If all else fails, I recommend ERCP with brush cytology and biopsy.

Extrahepatic bile duct cancer with mass (usually around the bile duct but occasionally intrabiliary as well) is best diagnosed by EUS FNA, as with pancreatic cancer. EUS visualizes the bile duct proximal to the hilum poorly, and detecting a mass is dependent on individual anatomy, size, and location of the lesion—in general, it is not helpful. EUS shows most of the left lobe of the liver but only a limited portion of the right liver. A previously placed stent may be helpful for localizing the site of the biliary mass. The yield of EUS FNA is quite low in patients with bile duct wall thickening only.

Therefore, ERCP, brush cytology, and/or biopsy are the only methods for diagnosing bile duct cancer in most patients, cancer located proximal to the hilum, or cancer without a discrete mass. The sensitivity of brush cytology is low at around 30% to 40% and can be improved by adding a second modality such as biopsy.[1] I think it is also reasonable to do multiple brushings (as in EUS FNA) during a single procedure to increase the diagnostic yield. Biliary biopsy can be performed under fluoroscopic guidance or under cholangioscopic guidance (Figure 25-3). Fluoroscopic-guided biopsy can be performed after sphincterotomy using conventional biopsy forceps but is limited by the inability to precisely target the biopsy sites with biopsies being done just distal to the stricture. Cholangioscopic biopsy can target the specific lesion (at least in theory), but all commercially available systems have limitations, especially in the intrahepatic ducts.

My approach to diagnosing a suspected bile duct is to start with EUS FNA to evaluate the extrahepatic system and eliminate pancreatic or ampullary cancer. If EUS FNA is negative for a mass but shows intrahepatic biliary dilation in the setting of a normal calib   ommon duct, then the lesion must be located in the hilum or proximal to it. I then

Figure 25-3. Pancreatoscopic visualization of an adenocarcinoma arising in the setting of IPMN.

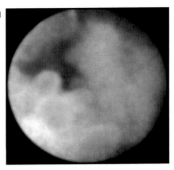

perform ERCP with brush cytology and biopsy of the biliary stricture. If everything is negative in a patient with high clinical suspicion, I perform cholangioscopy with directed biopsies. Unfortunately, the results may be negative even after repeated biopsies. In such cases, patients with high clinical suspicion and potentially resectable disease undergo an attempt at a surgical cure and the rest undergo close surveillance. I feel confident that a negative surveillance at 3 months almost always excludes the possibility of pancreatic cancer, but much longer follow-up is required in bile duct cancer and I generally recommend repeat EUS and possible ERCP every 3 months for 9 to 12 months before excluding cancer as a diagnosis.

References

1. Lee JG. Brush cytology and the diagnosis of pancreaticobiliary malignancy during ERCP. *Gastrointest Endosc.* 2006;63(1):78-80.
2. Chang KJ. State of the art lecture: endoscopic ultrasound (EUS) and FNA in pancreatico-biliary tumors. *Endoscopy.* 2006;38(Suppl 1):S56-S60.
3. Klapman JB, Chang KJ, Lee JG, Nguyen P. Negative predictive value of endoscopic ultrasound in a large series of patients with a clinical suspicion of pancreatic cancer. *Am J Gastroenterol.* 2005;100(12):2658-2661.
4. Root J, Nguyen N, Jones B, et al. Laparoscopic distal pancreatic resection. *Am Surg.* 2005;71(9):744-749.

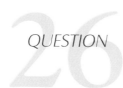

What Is the Role of Plastic Versus Metal Stents in Patients With Hilar Bile Duct Obstruction? Is There a Need for Bilateral Stenting for Malignant Hilar Obstruction?

Gregory Haber, MD

There are three principle issues when dealing with endoscopic management of malignant hilar obstruction: 1) establishing a diagnosis, 2) defining the anatomy, and 3) establishing the most effective drainage for palliation. Most of the published literature on this topic reviews retrospective experience from expert centers or reports prospective trials with the limitations inherent in the inclusion/exclusion criteria that define the trials. This presentation will address the issues listed above incorporating the collective published literature and personal experience.

Diagnosis of Malignant Hilar Obstruction

Obstruction at the hilum has a subtle early presentation as partial or unilobular blockage of the secondary or tertiary bile ducts, rarely causes specific diagnostic symptoms, and more often results in nonspecific complaints such as fatigue, malaise, or anorexia. The earliest clue to a problem localized to the hilum is an increase in cholestatic enzymes and, in particular, liver alkaline phosphatase or the finding of dilated intrahepatic bile ducts with a normal caliber common duct with/without a demonstrable mass lesion on screening transabdominal ultrasound.

The diagnosis may be considered in an asymptomatic individual during surveillance programs for conditions associated with an increased risk for cholangiocarcinoma:

* Primary sclerosing cholangitis (PSC)
* Hepatolithiasis
* Congenital hepatic fibrosis
* Clonorchiasis
* Opisthorchis viverrini
* Hepatitis C
* Choledochal cysts
* Anomalous pan-biliary anastomosis
* Thorium dioxide exposure

If there is suspected pathology, noninvasive modalities are clearly the first choice, but detailed imaging of the hilum is challenging for most cross sectional studies because the normal anatomy is complex and variants in ductal anatomy are common.

In expert hands employing micro bubble contrast agents (eg, Levovist [Schering AG, Berlin, Germany]), transabdominal ultrasound has been demonstrated to be as accurate as any other modality in outlining the level of the obstruction and the presence of a mass lesion. Correct prediction of resectability was 94% with an accuracy of 84% for T and N staging in a recent study reported from a Toronto group. These results, however, have only been described from expert centers and may not be achievable in most institutions.

The standard work-up now is magnetic resonance cholangiopancreatography (MRCP), which can outline the level of the obstruction and the presence of anomalous duct drainage. On the other hand, recognizing that primary bile duct cancer mostly infiltrates the submucosa and along perineural planes with a desmoplastic reaction, not surprisingly defining the level of obstruction by imaging techniques, underestimates the extent of the cancer. In that respect, complete evaluation for a potentially curable resection would necessitate a laborious and meticulous mapping by choledochoscopy via percutaneous transhepatic access to look for subtle endoscopic signs of tumor extension, such as vascular markings and minimal nodularity complemented with biopsy sampling. This approach is rarely employed in clinical practice, which reduces the chance of a Ro resection margin.

Computed tomography (CT) scanning is of little additional value in the assessment of primary bile duct cancers but may be helpful in evaluation of the other malignancies encountered such as pancreatic cancer, gallbladder cancer, hepatocellular carcinoma, metastatic nodal involvement, and lymphoma.

Examination of the hilum by endoscopic ultrasound is a difficult task and is useful only in a few expert centers. Anatomic mapping of the hilum and definition of mass lesions is the initial step in establishing a diagnosis, but tissue confirmation is desirable when feasible.

Pathologic confirmation is important given the occurrence of benign strictures isolated to the hilum that mimic cancer. A recent study reaffirms this problem, reporting on 49 patients with clinical and morphologic features of malignancy, increased carcinoembryonic antigen (CEA) and Ca 19-9, and undergoing surgery. Among these, 12 patients (24%) were found to have benign lesions, being an idiopathic fibrotic stricture in 10 and choledocholithiasis in 2. This is a well recognized clinical dilemma with several prior reports on this problem.

The endoscopic methods of tissue acquisition include aspiration of bile, brushing or biopsy directed by fluoroscopy at endoscopic retrograde cholangiopancreatography (ERCP), or needle sampling through a specialized catheter at ERCP or in a traditional manner using fine needle aspiration (FNA) with endoscopic ultrasound (EUS) guidance. The submucosal spread, the infiltrative pattern, and the desmoplastic reaction all conspire to make preoperative diagnosis difficult. The addition of tumor markers, including K-ras, CEA, telomerase, and aneuploidy, on flow cytometry may all be helpful, but none of these is entirely reliable with low specificity. In spite of the limitations, given the inaccuracy of imaging alone, a tissue diagnosis is often desirable but does require ERCP access.

Anatomic Definition of the Obstructed Hilum

The extent and location of the stricture are critical with respect to the possibility of resection and the planning of palliative stenting. MRCP is the best noninvasive and widely available modality for initial assessment, as noted previously. In general, surgical resection is predicated on the ability to preserve one lobe of the liver that has adequate function (ie, not cirrhotic) and an intact, noninvolved duct and branch of the portal vein and hepatic artery. The extent of ductal involvement has been classified according to Bismuth and Corlette and is critical to preoperative planning as well as the endoscopic approach to palliation. Type I is a cancer involving the common hepatic duct within 2 cm of the confluence but with communication of the main right and left hepatic ducts. Type II is occlusion at the hilum with involvement of the secondary branch ducts but without tertiary duct involvement. Type III is involvement of tertiary branch ducts limited to the right (IIIA) or left (IIIB) duct system. Type IV is involvement of tertiary branch ducts bilaterally. Type IV is unresectable and most Type III are similarly inoperable, whereas Type I and II are potentially resectable.

In the patient who is not an operative candidate, the stenting of Bismuth Type I is identical to obstruction at any level of the duct below the confluence, suitable for a single stent. The management of higher levels of obstruction is discussed following.

At ERCP, defining the duct morphology and the level of the stricture is mandatory in planning drainage. The usual patient position for ERCP (ie, the patient turned semi-prone) is inadequate for hilar pathology. The patient is best evaluated on his or her back, which helps to separate clearly the right and left duct systems with a fixed anteroposterior (AP) fluoroscopy head. A rotatable C-arm may accomplish the same projection for delineation of the ducts but is not always easy to maneuver bedside with most of the portable units in use. Either one of these approaches is essential to understanding the anatomy.

Endoscopic Palliation of Hilar Obstruction

The two questions that remain debatable are whether to use one stent or multiple stents for drainage and whether to use plastic or metal stents for this purpose.

The general principle is to drain all obstructed liver segments, which will maintain as much liver function as possible and prevent infection in a pool of static bile. While in theory this is desirable, the main drawback is the technical challenge this poses and the iatrogenic infection introduced with manipulation and contrast injection into ducts that remain undrained. Several early studies have shown high rates of cholangitis following ERCP in large part attributed to contamination of undrained segments.

The endoscopist must, therefore, decide if it is feasible to drain most of the obstructed ducts given his or her skill and experience, the morphology of the ducts as mapped out at MRCP, and whether there has been contamination of a segment from a prior ERCP or contrast injection at the initial ERCP.

Single lobe drainage has been validated by a trial in which approximately one-third of patients with hilar cancers were chosen for unilobular stenting based on initial MRCP imaging with intentional avoidance of contamination of the lobe for which drainage was not planned. This study showed reasonably effective drainage with a single stent and a very low rate of cholangitis. A subsequent prospective randomized Italian multi-center study showed no benefit of unilateral versus bilateral drainage, or vice-versa.

My own approach is to plan for bilateral drainage when possible and with potential advantages for the patient. This means that there is no atrophy of a lobe (ie, that it is still worth draining), that there is an accessible duct that is dilated and can accommodate a stent in both lobes, and that there is an option for complementary percutaneous drainage should it not be possible to drain a lobe filled with contrast. Given the technical challenges inherent in placement of multiple stents, these patients should be referred to an endoscopist experienced in managing this type of problem.

The following are the steps for bilateral plastic stenting:

1. Clearly delineate the anatomy.

2. Advance guidewires into each of the ducts to be drained before inserting the first stent.

3. Balloon dilate each stricture to be stented beforehand as these strictures are tight and do not easily accommodate two stents.

4. The first plastic stent inserted should be no larger than 8.5 Fr to allow passage alongside the wire in a scope channel of 4.2 mm or less and up to 11.5 Fr if a scope channel of 4.8 mm is being used.

5. In general, the toughest side to be stented should be done first because the second or third stent is usually tougher to advance.

6. The first stent should be left with a longer amount in the duodenum because it will be pushed further up when the second stent is advanced alongside it.

Bilateral metal stents share the same common approach up to the third step in the previous list. Subsequently, the left stent is inserted first with the ideal of leaving the lower end in the duodenum, depending on the length of the duct and the length of the stent. The right stent is then inserted with the lower end in the duodenum. This allows access to both stents for therapy for subsequent blockage. The alternative is to try to leave both ends of the stents at the same level of the duct so as to avoid the possibility that the expanded bottom of one stent does not preclude access to a stent above.

Metal stents can be inserted in parallel or alternatively in a Y configuration in which one stent traverses the wall of the other stent to enter the opposite lobe. This is achievable much more readily when there is a wide-open mesh, as is found with most of the newer nitinol stents. Some of these have been designed for this purpose and have a large window in the stent for passage of the second stent.

When single lobe drainage is planned, insertion of an uncoated metal stent is preferred to prolong patency and to avoid occlusion of branch ducts, which is more likely with a solid plastic stent. A small prospective randomized trial achieved equivalent palliation with fewer interventions when compared to the plastic arm of the trial.

Adjunctive Therapy

Additional tumor shrinkage can be achieved with photodynamic therapy as well as intraluminal brachytherapy, and these approaches are best applied bilaterally, which is another reason to attempt drainage of both liver lobes.

Conclusion

Endosopic palliation of malignant hilar obstruction remains one of the most challenging problems for the therapeutic endoscopist. There is no single correct approach for these patients, but judgment, skill, and experience are all essential for planning optimum care for these unfortunate individuals with a life expectancy of less than 1 year.

AN ELDERLY PATIENT WITH MULTIPLE MEDICAL PROBLEMS PRESENTED WITH ACUTE PANCREATITIS WITH STONES IN THE GALLBLADDER. HER LIVER FUNCTION STUDIES SHOW AN AST OF 90 AND AN ALT OF 85—BOTH ARE DECLINING. MRCP DID NOT DEMONSTRATE ANY CBD STONES OR DUCTAL DILATION. IS AN ERCP INDICATED?

Stuart Sherman, MD

This elderly patient has multiple medical problems and clearly has pancreatitis. In deciding whether an endoscopic retrograde cholangiopancreatography (ERCP) is indicated, I would want to know whether the pancreatitis is due to bile duct stones. Distinguishing biliary pancreatitis from other causes may be difficult, often requiring an extensive biochemical and radiologic evaluation. Finding gallbladder stones, as in this case, is suggestive but not conclusive of a biliary origin. A serum amylase level greater than 1000 IU/L should suggest a biliary tract origin although some overlap exists with other causes. A meta-analysis has suggested that a 3-fold or greater elevation in the alanine aminotransferase (ALT) in the presence of acute pancreatitis has a predictive value of 95% in diagnosing gallstone pancreatitis. Certainly, if one finds common duct stones on a radiologic imaging study, the diagnosis of stone-induced pancreatitis is near certain and ERCP indicated (unless a combined laparoscopic cholecystectomy and common duct exploration is possible). Magnetic resonance cholangiopancreatography (MRCP) has a sensitivity and specificity of detecting bile duct stones in the range of 90% to 100% and 92% to 100%, respectively. However, the sensitivity and specificity are reduced for small stones, which more commonly cause pancreatitis. Endoscopic ultrasound (EUS), when performed by experts, has comparable if not better accuracy in detecting bile duct stones than ERCP. When deciding whether or not to perform ERCP, single test results are less important than the constellation of findings that make up the overall clinical presentation. Remember, ERCP, as practiced currently, is used principally as a therapeutic modality to treat an anatomic obstruction as would be the case for bile duct stones. Based on the information provided, I can speculate that the patient likely has stone-induced pancreatitis but not certainly. Moreover, I have no clear evidence that there are stones in the bile duct by radiologic imaging tests and, as a result, no absolute reason to do an ERCP. Finally, the improving liver chemistries suggest that if indeed a stone was present in the bile duct, it likely has passed.

After I make a diagnosis of biliary pancreatitis, it is critical that I grade its severity and determine whether there is evidence of biliary tract obstruction or cholangitis. Addressing these issues will help to determine the necessity of ERCP. When cholangitis or jaundice complicates pancreatitis, the likelihood of finding an obstructing stone is increased. There are now four prospective randomized trials (three published as full papers and one as an abstract) that have attempted to define the role of early ERCP in gallstone pancreatitis. Two studies found an improved patient outcome from early ERCP in patients with predicted severe pancreatitis, one found no benefit from ERCP regardless of the pancreatitis severity, while the abstracted study found patients with mild and severe disease benefited. These four studies suggest that while certain patients with biliary pancreatitis benefit from early intervention with ERCP +/- biliary sphincterotomy and stone removal, others do not and may even suffer a worse outcome. At the State-of-the Science Conference on ERCP held in 2002, the conclusion drawn was that ERCP had a distinct role in the patient with severe biliary pancreatitis. In the case presented, it appears that the patient has mild gallstone pancreatitis, and I would advise against ERCP and recommend early laparoscopic cholecystectomy with intraoperative cholangiogram. However, there appear to be extenuating circumstances in that the patient has multiple medical problems and may be a poor surgical candidate. In such a patient, an ERCP should be considered as performing an empiric biliary sphincterotomy (even in the absence of finding bile duct stones) will prevent recurrent pancreatitis. If this approach is taken, what is the risk of leaving the gallbladder in situ? Older data suggested that the lifetime risk of developing a gallbladder complication (eg, acute cholecystitis) was about 10% to 20% in elderly patients. However, in a more recent randomized trial that compared laparoscopic cholecystectomy within 6 weeks of ERCP, sphincterotomy, and stone removal to a wait-and-see approach in surgically fit patients with known gallbladder stones, 47% of patients in the wait-and-see group developed biliary-related events compared to 2% in the cholecystectomy group. Thus, if the patient is felt to be a surgical candidate, ERCP should be avoided in favor of the cholecystectomy.

Conclusion

Assuming the magnetic resonance imaging (MRI)/MRCP shows no other pathology to explain the pancreatitis and the history and other laboratory tests are supportive of a gallstone origin, I would diagnose gallstone pancreatitis. An ERCP should not be done since the patient has a mild episode of pancreatitis and the improving liver tests suggest that the stone has passed. Assuming our patient is a surgical candidate, I would recommend laparoscopic cholecystectomy with intraoperative cholangiogram preferably during the current hospitalization. If the patient is felt to be a poor surgical candidate, then ERCP with empiric biliary sphincterotomy should be considered with the caveat that late gallbladder complications may occur.

References

1. Fogel EL, Sherman S. Acute biliary pancreatitis: when should the endoscopist intervene? *Gastroenterology.* 2003;125;229-235.
2. Kozarek R. Role of ERCP in acute pancreatitis. *Gastrointest Endosc.* 2002;56:S231-S236.
3. Sharma VK, Howden CW. Metaanalysis of randomized controlled trials of endoscopic retrograde cholangiography and endoscopic sphincterotomy for the treatment of acute biliary pancreatitis. *Am J Gastroenterol.* 1999;94:3211-3214.
4. Boerma D, Rauws EA, Keulemans YC, et al. Wait-and-see policy of laparoscopic cholecystectomy after endoscopic sphincterotomy for bile duct stones: a randomized trial. *Lancet.* 2002;360:761-765.

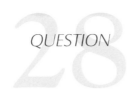

WHAT IS THE BEST APPROACH TO A PATIENT WITH A POST-LAP CHOLECYSTECTOMY BILE LEAK FROM THE CYSTIC DUCT STUMP, ABERRANT DUCTS, OR ASSOCIATED COMMON DUCT INJURY? IF INITIAL STENTING FAILS TO SEAL THE LEAK, WHAT ELSE CAN BE DONE ENDOSCOPICALLY?

Joseph Leung, MD, FRCP, FACP, FACG, FASGE

The best approach to a patient with a post-laparoscopic cholecystectomy bile leak is to confirm the site and (to some extent the severity) of the bile leakage at the time of endoscopic retrograde cholangiopancreatography (ERCP) (including, if necessary, the use of occlusion cholangiogram) in order to assess the outcome properly.

The management of a simple bile leakage from the cystic duct stump is by insertion of a 10 French (Fr) indwelling plastic stent with the proximal tip of the stent placed above the cystic duct insertion. This will ensure that the bile is collected by the stent. Although a biliary papillotomy alone has been reported to be effective, a papillotomy is not necessary for single stent placement, and this will avoid the risk of papillotomy-associated complications. Besides, a large papillotomy may predispose to upwards stent migration because the distal flap may not be able to hold the stent in place. Other reports have described the use of nasobiliary catheter drainage to decompress the biliary system, and this is an effective treatment for simple bile leak. However, an indwelling nasobiliary catheter causes patient discomfort and carries a risk of external bile loss and electrolyte imbalance. Proper anchorage of the nasobiliary catheter is necessary because the drain can be dislodged. Improper anchorage may predispose to unnecessary trauma to the nose.

Leak from the aberrant Luschka's ducts in the gallbladder bed can be controlled similarly with an indwelling biliary stent. In this situation, the leakage is more peripheral, and sometimes the intrabiliary pressure may be maintained if a small stent is used, thus predisposing to persistent leakage. Placement of a longer stent (close to the origin of the branch of the right hepatic duct that drains the aberrant ducts) is more helpful to divert the bile from the peripheral ducts. In some cases, I have resorted to inserting a nasobiliary catheter into the specific segment, draining the aberrant ducts in order to siphon the bile to promote healing of the bile leak.

In a more serious situation, such as injury to an aberrant duct draining part of the right lobe that arises from the cystic duct, injury can occur from inadvertent ligation and transaction, resulting in free bile leakage and a failure to demonstrate the leak on cholangiogram. Fortunately, this complication is not common. Management may involve interventional radiology with percutaneous transhepatic cholangiogram to determine the exact site of ductal injury and leakage. In a complete transaction, the injury may require a surgical bilioenteric anastomosis to control the leak.

Associated Common Duct Injury

If the presence of a bile leak is associated with common bile duct injury, it is important to define the location and extent of the injury. The most common cause of ductal injury is due to excess cautery or thermal injury often as a result of hemostasis. This may leave a vent in the bile duct wall as a result of tissue necrosis. Injury may be a result of clip injury to the bile duct. In both cases, there is a risk of late bile duct stenosis or stricture formation.

In the management of the bile leak, it is necessary to seal off the area of ductal injury. Simply providing drainage distally may not be sufficient to control the bile leak. I recommend negotiating the ductal injury area with a guidewire and inserting a 10-Fr stent across the leak. In doing so, the indwelling stent provides drainage of bile and helps to seal off the leak. At the same time, the stent provides splintage of the damaged bile duct and promotes healing. In the event of a late ductal stricture, access is maintained across the stricture, which will facilitate subsequent endoscopic therapy. Balloon dilation is not recommended in the immediate postsurgical period even in the presence of possible stenosis to avoid extending the ductal injury and leak. Partial clip injury to the bile duct may create a stenosis, and it may be necessary to resort to percutaneous transhepatic manipulation to try and cross the area of injury and to loosen the clip. Placement of a stent across the area of duct injury promotes healing and prevents further leakage. If necessary, balloon dilation and prolonged stenting may be required later to treat the bile duct stenosis.

Persistent bile leakage may be a result of large area of damage to the bile duct wall predisposing to the leakage. The relative discrepancy between the size of the leak and lumen of the stent may be one reason for persist leakage. If necessary, a papillotomy is performed and multiple stents are inserted into the bile duct across the area of the leak to divert all the bile back into the duodenum.

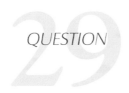
WHAT SHOULD MY RESPONSE BE TO A SURGEON WHO DEMANDS THAT I DO PRELAPAROSCOPIC CHOLECYSTECTOMY ERCP ON ALL OF HIS GALLSTONE PATIENTS?

John G. Lee, MD

The answer is no since endoscopic retrograde cholangiopancreatogram (ERCP) is never indicated in 100% of any group of patients. However, the response is more complicated to a surgeon who wants preoperative ERCP in most of his or her patients with gallstones and depends on the reason why the surgeon wants the ERCP. Some examples are given as follows:

*   The surgeon believes that most of the patients have high probability of having common duct stones and wants them removed before laparoscopic cholecystectomy. This is an appropriate indication, and routine ERCP should be performed. However, the prevalence of unsuspected common bile duct stone is around 5% to 15% in patients undergoing laparoscopic cholecystectomy, so this is an unlikely scenario.

*   The surgeon wants routine ERCP to delineate the biliary anatomy due to lack of experience performing laparoscopic cholecystectomy. This may have been an acceptable indication when laparoscopic cholecystectomy was developed but is not an acceptable indication for ERCP.

*   Probably the most common reason that a surgeon wants routine preoperative ERCP is that he or she does not have confidence in your ability to perform postoperative ERCP and stone extraction in a timely and successfully manner and wants to avoid a second surgical common duct exploration (which also means that he or she does not want to remove the stone laparoscopically). The success rate of ERCP and stone extraction should be very close to 100% (but probably never 100% in any center) in

Figure 29-1. (A) Postoperative ERCP shows multiple large stones. (B) Sphincterotomy and balloon dilation using a 14-mm balloon was done. (C) All the stones were removed intact without lithotripsy. Note the 14-mm biliary orifice (arrow). (D) Final cholangiogram shows stone clearance and air in the biliary tree.

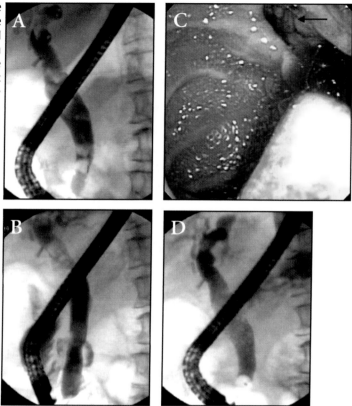

referral centers and should be at least in the high 80% in nonreferral centers (Figure 29-1). The success rate of ERCP is not entirely dependent on the ability of the endoscopist. For example, urgent ERCP may not be possible or very difficult in some hospitals, or some smaller hospitals may not even have emergency ERCP coverage. Again, I think the demand to perform routine preoperative ERCP will be relatively uncommon in centers with readily available good ERCP capabilities because most surgeons already recognize it. If you feel the surgeon is misinformed or falsely pessimistic, then you could try to educate him or her about your skills, training, experience, and outcome of ERCP. Round-the-clock availability of a tertiary care center with a proven track record for performing successful ERCP in a timely, customer service-oriented manner should also help allay the surgeon's concern about having to perform second surgery after failed ERCP and reduce the request for routine preoperative ERCP.

Preoperative ERCP should be only considered in patients with cholangitis, jaundice, elevated liver tests, imaging showing bile duct stones, or worsening gallstone pancreatitis.[1,2] Preoperative ERCP should also be done as dictated by the surgical plan, for example in patients with anticipated anatomical problems such as prior biliary tract surgery (Figure 29-2). Preoperative ERCP is not indicated in patients with suspected but unconfirmed common duct stone or resolving jaundice because magnetic resonance cholangiopancreatography (MRCP), or better yet, endoscopic ultrasound (EUS) can be as accurate and significantly less risky compared to ERCP.

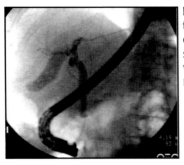

Figure 29-2. Preoperative abdominal ultrasound and computed tomography (CT) showed a liver mass in a patient who presented with suspected gallstones. EUS did not show a common duct stone but what looked like an intrahepatic gallbladder. ERCP was performed to outline the biliary anatomy to facilitate laparoscopic cholecystectomy, which was performed successfully.

The need for preoperative ERCP is less straight forward in patients without one of the above clear cut indications and depends primarily on the risk of finding an unsuspected stone at the time of laparoscopic cholecystectomy and the surgical and endoscopic expertise. Patients with low risk of common duct stone (<10%) do not need any tests; patients with risk of stone, >11% but <55%, should undergo EUS, and patients with risk >55%, should undergo preoperative ERCP according to one decision analysis.[3] I would modify this recommendation with the following changes: substitute high-quality MRCP for EUS if it is not available and always perform EUS before ERCP unless the patient is jaundiced, has cholangitis, worsening pancreatitis, or known common duct stones. We perform EUS immediately prior to ERCP in about two-thirds of patients scheduled for ERCP and forego the procedure if EUS is negative. In my clinical experience, EUS is much more sensitive than ERCP for detecting common duct stones, especially small ones, and should be used as the definitive test rather than ERCP. Preoperative biliary imaging is superfluous if every patient undergoes intraoperative cholangiogram and laparoscopic stone extraction (a highly unlikely scenario).

In summary, I recommend considering preoperative ERCP only in patients with jaundice, cholangitis, elevated liver tests, known common duct stone, or worsening gallstone pancreatitis. All others should undergo EUS if available or MRCP rather than ERCP with ERCP and stone extraction reserved only for patients with documented common duct stones.

References

1. Adler DG, Baron TH, Davila RE, et al. ASGE guideline: the role of ERCP in diseases of the biliary tract and the pancreas. *Gastrointest Endosc.* 2005;62(1):1-8.
2. National Institutes of Health. Endoscopic retrograde cholangiopancreatography (ERCP) for diagnosis and therapy. *NIH Consens Statement Online.* 2002;19(1):1-23.
3. Sahai AV, Mauldin PD, Marsi V, et al. Bile duct stones and laparoscopic cholecystectomy: a decision analysis to assess the roles of intraoperative cholangiography, EUS, and ERCP. *Gastrointest Endosc.* 1999;49(3 Pt 1):334-343.

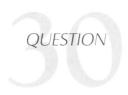
WHAT SHOULD BE THE SEQUENCE OF INVESTIGATIONS FOR A PATIENT WITH RECURRENT, UNEXPLAINED PANCREATITIS?

Stuart Sherman, MD

Determining the cause of acute pancreatitis is not usually difficult. Alcohol and gallstones are the two most common etiologies and account for 60% to 90% of cases. Alcoholism is diagnosed by history and gallstones by a combination of demographic characteristics, laboratory findings, and radiographic imaging studies. In patients in whom acute pancreatitis is due to hypertiglyceridemia, hypercalcemia, drug reactions, trauma, surgery, endoscopic retrograde cholangiopancreatography (ERCP), etc, the relationship of the episode of pancreatitis to the cause is usually clear. Nevertheless, a cause for the pancreatitis will not be identified in 10% to 30% of patients after a careful history, physical examination, laboratory studies, transabdominal ultrasound, and computed tomography (CT) scanning. These patients are conventionally classified as having idiopathic acute pancreatitis (IAP). Patients with recurrent episodes of IAP are diagnosed with idiopathic acute recurrent pancreatitis (IARP). Some authorities reserve the terms *IAP* and *IARP* for those patients who remain undiagnosed after a more detailed endoscopic (ERCP with manometry, endoscopic ultrasound [EUS]), radiologic (eg, magnetic resonance cholangiopancreatography [MRCP]), laboratory (eg, for autoimmune pancreatitis), and genetic evaluation and use the term *unexplained pancreatitis* prior to the more intensive investigation.

There are two major concerns that prompt the physician to do a more intensive evaluation of the patient with acute pancreatitis in whom no obvious cause is determined. The first is that the patient may have an underlying disease that will predispose him or her to further attacks of acute pancreatitis unless the cause is identified and adequately treated. The second concern is that the pancreatitis is due to a neoplastic condition. There are no standardized evidence-based algorithms to guide us, and the approach to the evaluation is often center specific and in part related to the expertise available. After a single episode of unexplained pancreatitis, the role of invasive evaluation with ERCP is unsettled but often limited to patients in whom there is suspicion of bile duct stones or a neoplastic process. I remain concerned about this approach in patients older than 40 years (when neoplasia becomes more common) because the "standard evaluation" might miss an unsuspected neoplastic process, such as an intraductal papillary mucinous neoplasm (IPMN). With the more widespread availability and expertise in EUS and MRCP/magnetic resonance imaging (MRI), ERCP is often relegated to patients found to have a treatable endoscopic disease (eg, bile duct stones, pancreas divisum) or those found to have normal EUS and/or MRCP/MRI where further endoscopic investigation is warranted (eg, evaluation by sphincter of Oddi manometry [SOM]).

I am asked to provide a sequence of investigations for the patient presenting with IARP. I will make the assumption that a standard evaluation has been done as described previously and has been negative, including repeat triple phase abdominal CT scan with pancreatic protocol and transabdominal ultrasound (US) when the gallbladder is in situ. It is important to stratify patients by their age and gallbladder status to help direct your approach. Certainly younger patients are less likely to have a neoplastic process, and those with the gallbladder in situ may have microlithiasis as an explanation for the pancreatitis. Given the results of two frequently cited studies suggesting that microlithiasis (often defined as stones <3 mm in diameter and frequently missed on transabdominal US) was the cause for the pancreatitis in 67% to 74% of patients, some authorities advocate empiric cholecystectomy. Other studies and my own experience refute this high prevalence of microlithiasis, and as a result, I do not support this approach unless there is evidence of stone-related disease by bile sampling, transabdominal US, or EUS. EUS is perhaps the most sensitive way to detect biliary sludge and microlithiasis.

My initial work-up will include repeat laboratory testing consisting of serum triglyceride and calcium levels. It is critical to try to obtain the results of these tests during the attack as they may be normal or near normal when the patient is asymptomatic. Although controversial, I will usually evaluate the patient's cystic fibrosis transmembrane conductance regulator (CFTR) gene, given the relatively high prevalence of cystic fibrosis gene mutations in patients with IARP (around 20% versus 3% in the normal population without pancreatitis). However, a positive result will not preclude further investigation. Unless there is some suggestion that at least one family member had an episode of pancreatitis, I do not routinely assess for other known genetic causes of pancreatitis (PRSS1 gene and SPINK1 gene) because of the low yield and high cost. Serologic (eg, serum IgG 4 level) and confirmatory testing and/or therapy (eg, pancreatic biopsy or corticosteroids) for autoimmune pancreatitis are done in the appropriate setting when supported by consistent clinical, radiographic, and ERCP findings. My recommendations, as to the next test(s), are based on having available expertise in both EUS and MRI/MRCP. In many respects, EUS and secretin-enhanced MRCP/MRI are duplicative and may not be additive. EUS can better assess for gallbladder pathology (duodenal collection of bile after cholecystokinin stimulation can be done simultaneously if the EUS fails to demonstrate gallbladder pathology), small bile duct stones, chronic pancreatitis, and pancreatic/peripancreatic neoplasia, but secretin-enhanced MRCP/MRI gives very detailed images of

Table 30-1
Idiopathic Acute Recurrent Pancreatitis—Diagnostic Yield of ERCP, Sphincter of Oddi Manometry, and Bile Microscopy*

Diagnosis	Number Abnormal
Sphincter of Oddi dysfunction	179 (34%)
Pancreas divisum	70 (13%)
Pancreatic or papillary tumor	46 (9%)
Gallbladder or duct stones	37 (7%)
Pancreatic duct stricture/chronic pancreatitis	37 (7%)
Choledochocele	12 (2%)
Total abnormal	381/522 (73%)

*4 selected series of 522 patients

the pancreatic duct and biliary tree anatomy. In my experience, secretin enhancement is necessary to get the best quality images of the pancreatic duct. Because of the increasing concern for neoplasia with age, I will usually recommend an EUS for patients 40 years or older. The diagnostic yield of EUS in IARP varies from 32% to 88%. There are limited data addressing the yield of secretin-enhanced MRCP/MRI in this setting, but I suspect that a good quality study would provide nearly equivalent diagnostic accuracy as an ERCP (MRCP/MRI will often miss ampullary tumors and IPMNs particularly in normal diameter pancreatic ducts). In younger patients, I will often obtain a secretin-enhanced MRI/MRCP before considering a more invasive assessment with ERCP. ERCP should be reserved for those IARP patients who either have a normal EUS and/or secretin-stimulated MRI/MRCP or where the disease identified is treatable by endoscopic methods (eg, pancreas divisum). Since sphincter of Oddi dysfunction (SOD) is the most common cause of IARP identified in ERCP series, the ability to perform SOM at the time of ERCP is mandatory. There is no role for diagnostic ERCP in this setting, and the endoscopist should have expertise in managing the diseases uncovered such as pancreas divisum, SOD choledochocele, and pancreatic strictures. It is critical that a detailed pancreatogram be done at ERCP and high-resolution fluoroscopy be available. I have seen many patients with reportedly normal pancreatic ducts on EUS, MRCP, and/or prior ERCP but have very subtle cast-like filling defects in a normal diameter pancreatic duct, which is highly suggestive of an IPMN. ERCP clearly plays an important role in the management of patients with IARP. In this setting, the reported diagnostic yield of ERCP, ± SOM, ± bile microscopy varies from 38% to 79%, and the overall yield is influenced by the presence or absence of the gallbladder and referral bias. Table 30-1 presents a compilation of 4 series evaluating the yield of ERCP and ancillary procedures. The large majority of diseases uncovered are treatable by endoscopic or surgical techniques.

References

1. Wilcox CM, Varadarjulu S, Eloubeidi M. Role of endoscopic evaluation in idiopathic pancreatitis: a systematic review. *Gastrointest Endosc.* 2006;63;1037-1045.
2. Levy MJ, Geenen JE. Idiopathic acute recurrent pancreatitis. *Am J Gastroenterol.* 2001;96:2540-2555.
3. Evans WB, Draganov P. Is empiric cholecystectomy a reasonable treatment option for idiopathic acute pancreatitis. *Nat Clin Prac Gastroenterol Hepatol.* 2006;3:356-357.
4. Steinberg WM, Chari ST, Forsmark CE, et al. Controversies in clinical pancreatology: management of acute idiopathic recurrent pancreatitis. *Pancreas.* 2003;27:103-117.
5. Kaw M, Brodmerkel GJ. ERCP, biliary crystal analysis, and sphincter of Oddi manometry in idiopathic pancreatitis. *Gastrointest Endosc.* 2002;55:157-162.

I Have a Patient With Biliary-Type Pain but No Other Evidence of Bile Duct Disease (Normal Diameter Duct on Ultrasound, Normal Liver Function Tests). How Should Such a Patient Be Managed?

Martin L. Freeman, MD

Right upper quadrant (RUQ) pain syndrome is most common in women, particularly those who are young to middle-aged. The first question we should ask is whether the gallbladder is intact. Our first efforts should be to thoroughly investigate whether there is any evidence of gallbladder disease. Computed tomography (CT) scan is generally performed to look for structural abnormalities but is generally negative. A high-quality RUQ ultrasound should be done. If there is any evidence of gallbladder sludge or stone disease, it is reasonable to offer laparoscopic cholecystectomy. If negative, then a cholecystokinin (CCK)-stimulated hydroxyindole diaminoacetic acid (HIDA) nuclear medicine scan can be done to look for a diminished ejection fraction, indicative of "gallbladder dyskinesia." If abnormal, then cholecystectomy can be recommended. Although I also recommend this approach, I counsel patients that there is about a 50% chance or less of clinical improvement and very limited supporting data. If the CCK HIDA scan is negative, I recommend endoscopic ultrasound, which may find subtle evidence of gallbladder sludge, chronic pancreatitis, ductal abnormalities, or occasionally some other surprise—I once found pericardial effusions suggestive of pericarditis not suspected by any other test. In very rare circumstances, I will recommend consideration of empirical cholecystectomy in the absence of any gallbladder disease even by all of the above tests. I do not recommend endoscopic retrograde cholangiopancreatography (ERCP) or sphincter of Oddi manometry (SOM) for unexplained RUQ pain in patients with intact gallbladders.

The next and more difficult question is what to do if there is persistent recurrent RUQ pain after the gallbladder has been removed. Then the differential narrows down to very rare structural disorders such as bile duct stones, which are almost never found, motility disorders such as gastroparesis, "visceral hyperalgesia," peritoneal adhesions, minimal change chronic pancreatitis, or sphincter of Oddi dysfunction (SOD). Where to go next is highly dependent on clinical suspicion and, frankly, is mostly driven by the beliefs of the physician seeing the patient and belief in the existence in the various diagnostic entities. First and foremost is to take a careful history. Is the pain consistent and reproducible? Is there any precipitating factor, such as eating fatty foods? Does movement exacerbate the pain? If so, it may be suggestive of a musculoskeletal rather than a visceral disorder. Is the pain an isolated symptom or is there nausea, vomiting, or postprandial bloating, which may suggest gastroparesis? Many patients have multiple other pain syndromes, such as migraine headaches and fibFromyalgia. It is also important to document liver and pancreatic chemistries during or after pain attacks on at least three separate occasions, if possible. Abnormal results may only occur sporadically after pain attacks, which may point to a biliary or pancreatic cause. Very occasionally, laparoscopy can be considered to look for "adhesions," but this almost never yields results. Often, empirical trials of anti-spasmodics or antidepressants are given but seldom yield a satisfactory response.

If I am still suspecting a structural or functional cause, I generally proceed with endo-scopic ultrasound to look for subtle evidence of biliary or pancreatic disease. A number of these patients will have equivocal or suggestive evidence of small-duct chronic pancreati-tis, with 3 to 5 out of 9 possible criteria. The significance of such findings is debatable but may be the only evidence of chronic pancreatitis. If EUS is done before any kind of inter-vention, the results are interpretable and will not represent iatrogenic artifact of ERCP or pancreatic stents. I also generally obtain secretin-enhanced MRCP to look for structural abnormalities such as pancreas divisum or abnormal augmentation of pancreatic duct with secretin stimulation. Very rarely, MRCP will reveal biliary tract disease such as a choledochal cyst. It also will provide a road map, particularly of the pancreatic duct, that will become critical if ERCP with SOM is contemplated.

Whether to proceed with ERCP with SOM is the most difficult and controversial deci-sion. It depends in the physician's belief in SOD. It is widely believed that likelihood of SOD and chance of response are mostly determined by the presence or absence of abnor-mal liver chemistries or dilated bile duct—the so-called "Milwaukee" criteria dividing patients into Type I (dilated bile duct and abnormal liver chemistries), Type II (either but not both), or Type III (neither present, such as our case discussed here), with probability of existence and response to sphincterotomy descending from high to none from Type I to Type III.[1] This construct is based on the concept that SOD is a biliary disease. We now know that if it exists, it involves both the pancreatic and biliary sphincter (Figure 31-1).[2] Patients may respond to pancreatic sphincterotomy in addition to biliary sphincterotomy where biliary sphincterotomy alone generally fails to improve symptoms (Figure 31-2). Recent data from our center suggest that, in fact, outcomes of dual biliary and pancreatic sphincterotomy have little relation to Milwaukee type but rather are dependent on clini-

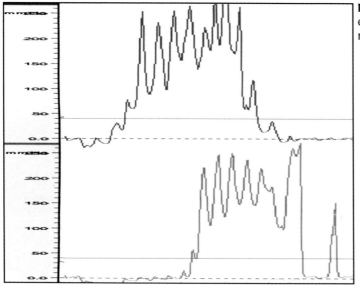

Figure 31-1. SOM showing elevated basal pressure (>40 mm).

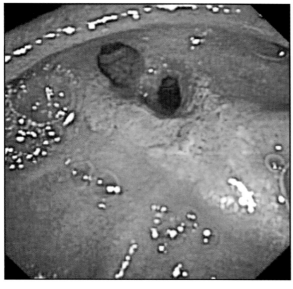

Figure 31-2. Complete pancreatic and biliary sphincterotomies at follow-up.

cal factors indicative of a more global dysfunction, such as dependence on narcotic analgesics or the presence of gastroparesis.[3] In addition, findings at pancreatic manometry are predictive. I no longer believe that the Milwaukee classification is particularly relevant to outcomes of suspected SOD. My views are different from the generally held opinion,[4] but I believe that further research will bear out the importance of the "bigger picture" beyond simple indicators of biliary obstruction.

We do know that ERCP of any kind is highly risky in patients with suspected SOD, and that post-ERCP pancreatitis can be greatly reduced by placement of a temporary, small caliber pancreatic stent, which is now considered almost mandatory in such patients (Figures 31-3 and 31-4).[5]

Figure 31-3. Guidewire in pancreatic duct after biliary sphincterotomy.

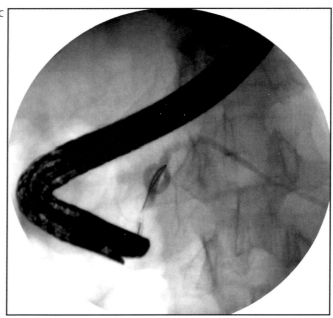

Figure 31-4. Pancreatic stent placed to reduce risk of post-ERCP pancreatitis, draining pancreatic juice.

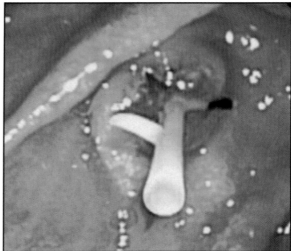

So what would I do in a patient postcholecystectomy with intractable, recurrent RUQ pain suspected to be of biliary or pancreatic origin with no objective evidence of biliary disease? After EUS and secretin MRCP, assuming they are normal or show nonspecific changes, discuss the risk/benefit of ERCP with possible dual biliary and pancreatic sphincterotomy depending on manometric findings. I tell patients that the outcome depends on the other factors (young age, narcotic dependence, and/or gastroparesis) that lower the expected response dramatically; if none of these negative predictors are present, and pancreatic manometry is found to be abnormal, then response rates are about 60%. I quote a risk of mild post-ERCP pancreatitis of about 15% with a small but real chance (about 1/200 to 1/300) of severe or even life-threatening complications. I tell patients that some major centers do not believe in this entity. I let the patient decide whether to proceed.

At this point, about half of patients I see wish to pursue ERCP. I do ERCP under general anesthesia, for safety and comfort. I start with aspirated pancreatic sphincter manometry. If that is abnormal, I proceed with biliary and pancreatic sphincterotomy. If pancreatic manometry is normal, I perform biliary manometry. If agreed in advance, in selective cases, I may perform biliary sphincterotomy without a manometry but not pancreatic sphincterotomy. Regardless of what type of maneuvers are performed, I place a small caliber (currently 4 French (Fr) 2 cm, single inner flanged soft-material) pancreatic stent to reduce risk. I admit all these patients for inpatient observation, keep them NPO (given nothing by mouth), medicate pain and nausea, which often occurs independent of development of pancreatitis, and do not feed them until amylase or lipase is checked and is less than 2 to 3 times normal or the patient feels fine. The pancreatic stent is always documented to pass or is removed within 2 weeks.

Some patients with SOD clearly respond to endoscopic intervention while others do not. Our response rates for Type III SOD are not significantly different than response rates for Type I or II, at about 60%.[3] Whether any treatment is truly effective will only be answered by a randomized, controlled trial, which is currently being planned by Dr. Cotton and colleagues and funded by the National Institutes of Health (NIH).

ERCP for abdominal pain syndromes in the absence of clear-cut biliary obstructive disease should only be performed at major centers with an extensive interest, high degree of endoscopic expertise in SOM and pancreatic as well as biliary endotherapy, and particularly with placement of small caliber pancreatic stents with near 100% success regardless of the pancreatic ductal anatomy. Otherwise, the risk of ERCP clearly outweighs the benefit.

References

1. Sherman S. What is the role of ERCP in the setting of abdominal pain of pancreatic or biliary origin (suspected sphincter of Oddi dysfunction)? *Gastrointest Endosc.* 2002;56:S258-S266.
2. Aymerich RR, Prakash C, Aliperti G. Sphincter of oddi manometry: is it necessary to measure both biliary and pancreatic sphincter pressures? *Gastrointest Endosc.* 2000;52:183-186.
3. Freeman ML, Gill M, Overby C, Cen Y. Predictors of outcomes after biliary and pancreatic sphincterotomy for sphincter of Oddi dysfunction. *J Clin Gastroentero.* 2007;41:94-102.
4. Cohen S, Bacon BR, Berlin JA, et al. National Institutes of Health State-of-the-Science Conference Statement: ERCP for diagnosis and therapy, January 14-16, 2002. *Gastrointest Endosc.* 2002;56:803-809.
5. Freeman ML, Guda NM. Prevention of post-ERCP pancreatitis: a comprehensive review. *Gastrointest Endosc.* 2004;59:845-864.

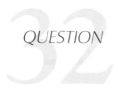

HOW CAN WE ACCURATELY DETERMINE THE APPROPRIATE LENGTH OF THE STENT TO USE IN A PATIENT WITH A BILE DUCT STRICTURE?

Joseph Leung, MD, FRCP, FACP, FACG, FASGE, and Erina Foster, MD

By definition, the length of a plastic stent refers to the shaft of the stent that traverses a bile duct stricture and is often indicated by the separation between the proximal and distal side flaps. The flaps are used to resist stent migration. For pigtail stent design, the length is defined as the separation between the pigtails. When stents were first invented, they were used mainly in patients with malignant bile duct obstruction. Indications for biliary stenting have now expanded to include benign strictures and large bile duct stones.

In the management of a bile duct stricture, it is generally accepted that the proximal flap be placed about 1 cm above the upper level of the obstruction (in order to allow for possible tumor extension) and with the distal flap placed at the level of the papilla. In determining the appropriate length of a biliary stent, it is important to define the upper level of the stricture and if there is involvement of the right and left hepatic ducts at the bifurcation.

Different methods are available for measuring the length of a stent. A conventional radiograph has an average magnification factor of up to 30%, and the distance between the papilla and the upper level of the stricture as measured on the cholangiogram should be corrected for magnification, then add 1 cm to give the length of the stent.

An indirect measurement of the stent length can be made by comparing the estimated separation between the upper level of the bile duct obstruction and the papilla with the diameter of the duodenoscope (Figure 32-1). The diameter of endoscopic retrograde cholangiopancreatography (ERCP) scopes vary between 11 and 13 mm. The separation between the papilla and the upper level of the stricture can be estimated by the number

Figure 32-1. (A) The length of the stent is denoted by the separation between the proximal and distal flaps. (B) It can be estimated with reference to the diameter of the duodenoscope, either on fluoroscopy or on a plain radiograph.

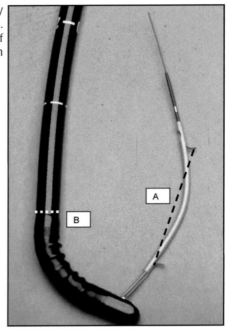

of scope diameters between the two points. With an adequate cholangiogram, locating the upper level of the stricture is often easy, whereas locating the exact level of the papilla could be more difficult. The position of the papilla can be determined by up-angulation of the scope tip against the papilla. No correction for magnification is necessary because the scope is in the same plane as the bile duct. It is, however, important to realize that the lower end of the column of contrast may not represent the true papillary orifice because there is a variable length of the intraduodenal papilla and sphincter that may not be filled by contrast.

Direct measurement of this separation can be obtained by using a guidewire and a catheter with a radiopaque tip or papillotome. Deep cannulation is achieved, leaving either a catheter or papillotome above the stricture. The guidewire is pulled back until the tip is at the upper level of the stricture as seen on fluoroscopy. The guidewire is then pulled back until the tip is seen emerging from the bile duct within the catheter lumen at the papilla. The length of guidewire pulled out is measured at the proximal end of the catheter or papillotome at the injection port to give a direct measurement of the separation and, thus, the length of stent to be used. An alternative is to pull back a catheter or papillotome over a deeply placed guidewire until the fluoroscopic tip or marker is seen at the level of the papilla. Again, the distance traveled by the catheter or papillotome is measured at the level of the biopsy valve. This will give an accurate measurement of the separation between the upper level of the stricture and papilla and thus the length of stent to be used.

For those who use the traditional three-layer system (guidewire, inner catheter, and pusher) for stent placement, an estimate of the stent length can be done by using the inner catheter with radiopaque ring markers (such as the Wilson Cook stenting system, [Wilson Cooke, Winston-Salem, NC]) to do the measurement. The inner catheter is positioned across the stricture and the separation between the papilla can be estimated by referencing the separation of the markers. However, with the new stenting (eg, OASIS, Wilson Cook) systems in which the inner catheter and pusher are combined into one, a proper length stent has to be chosen and loaded onto the delivery system prior to insertion. This makes the use of inner catheter with markers useless for stent measurement.

Another way of estimating the length of stent is using devices containing markers that have a fixed separation and comparing it against the separation between the papilla and the stricture. This is, however, more difficult as the device has to be moved and there is no fixed point of reference. Such devices include dilation balloons with ring markers or the flexible tip of a cytology brush.

Special Considerations

If the stricture is located in the distal bile duct, a short stent may result in easy dislocation. In general, straight stents have curved or angulated shapes to prevent stent migration. A short stent placed in the distal bile duct is prone to migration because it may not conform to the shape of the bile duct. We recommend the use of a slightly longer stent or sometimes shaping the stent so that it conforms to the contour of the bile duct and provides better anchorage. As a general rule, for distal bile duct strictures, we use a 7- to 8-cm stent. For patients with mid common bile duct (CBD) obstruction, a 10-cm stent is used and a longer stent is necessary if the stricture is close to the bifurcation.

For strictures located at the bifurcation, it is important to determine if the right and left hepatic system are obstructed separately. If so, we may need to consider stenting of both the right and left hepatic ducts. For drainage of the right side, it is possible to place a longer stent such as a 12-cm stent, leaving the tip in one of the branch ducts, and allow bile to flow in a retrograde manner into the anchoring segment and then down the stent.

For a left hepatic duct stricture, it is much more convenient to use the 15-cm stent, leaving a good portion of the stent within the bile duct. It is not uncommon to see kinking or buckling of a straight stent when it is deployed in the left hepatic duct. This is due to the configuration of the stent, which usually conforms to the contour of the common hepatic and the right intrahepatic system. We advocate the use of the "left hepatic duct" stent, which is shaped like a Z, allowing the proximal part of the stent to stay within the left hepatic duct and the remaining shaft of the stent conforming to the mid and distal portion of the bile duct.

Reference

1. Leung JW. Fundamentals of ERCP. In: Cotton P, Leung JW, eds. *Advanced Digestive Endoscopy—ERCP*. Boston, MA: Blackwell Publishing; 2005.

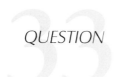
I HAVE DIFFICULTY CONTROLLING THE DIRECTION OF A BILIARY PAPILLOTOMY. ANY TRICKS TO IMPROVE THE RESULTS?

Joseph Leung, MD, FRCP, FACP, FACG, FASGE, and Erina Foster, MD

Before we discuss how to improve a biliary papillotomy, we have to understand the basic factors that determine the success of a biliary papillotomy.

The Perfect Axis

It is well recognized that the "perfect" axis for a biliary papillotomy is along the so-called 11 to 12 o'clock direction. However, experts' consensus defines the "perfect axis" as the longitudinal axis of the distal (intraduodenal) bile duct and the papilla, and the cut should be conducted along this axis rather than just the 12 o'clock direction as seen on the endoscopy screen (Figure 33-1). Some experts recommend aligning this axis with the 12 o'clock direction by manipulating the duodenoscope before performing the cut. It is also important to understand that this "perfect" axis will not change since this is part of the underlying anatomy, but the alignment of the scope with the papilla may change as a result of a displaced papilla or a change in the scope tip position. It is, therefore, important to recognize the axis before starting the papillotomy. With this in mind, it may be easier to understand how to improve a biliary papillotomy.

A number of factors can alter the perfect axis. Most of these are anatomical, including a periampullary diverticulum or diverticula, which tend to distort the axis of the papilla and distal bile duct. In this situation, the distal bile duct axis may fall on the edge of the diverticulum. Air insufflation distends the diverticulum and may further distort the axis, making alignment of the papillotome more difficult. An impacted stone may alter the position of the papilla, but it is more likely to make the axis more obvious due to the

Figure 33-1. (A) Consensus of a panel of 27 expert biliary endoscopists suggests the "perfect" axis of biliary sphincterotomy is along the 11 to 12 o'clock direction (ie, axis of distal bile duct and papilla), and (B) not just 12 o'clock direction seen on endoscopy screen. Also, the direction can change with scope position but the axis does not.

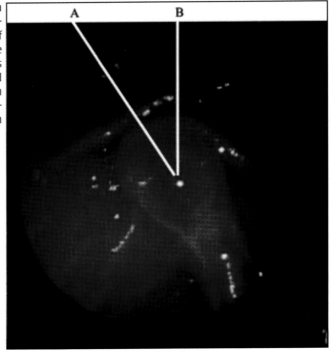

bulging distal bile duct. Prior duodenal ulcer disease, chronic pancreatitis, surgery, or an underlying head of pancreas tumor may cause deformity of the duodenum and, thus, difficulty in manipulating and positioning the endoscope, especially when pulling back the scope into a short scope position. This deformity also limits scope tip movement and, as a result, causes difficulty in achieving and maintaining a good position for papillotomy.

A second important factor that determines the direction of the cut is the papillotome itself.

Most papillotome wire tends to deviate toward the right side when tension or traction is applied to the cutting wire. This may be due to the fact that opening of the scope channel and elevator is located off to the right side of the tip of the duodenoscope. To some extent, this deviation can be overcome by adjusting the scope tip position in order to maintain proper alignment with the papilla during cutting. Sometimes, it is useful to consider shaping the papillotome (Figure 33-2) (by rotating the tip of the papillotome so that the wire is positioned almost 90 degrees to the left of the catheter and then curling the tip of the papillotome between the thumb, index, and middle fingers). In doing so, the wire is aligned along the left side of the catheter, and when traction is applied, the cutting wire tends to stay in a more neutral position. Changing the tension of the wire can also alter the wire position and thus its alignment/contact with the papilla. Sometimes, it may be necessary to over-relax the wire to allow it to stay in a more neutral position. Pushing the scope further into the duodenum and achieving a semi-long position may change the cutting wire position into better alignment with the papilla.

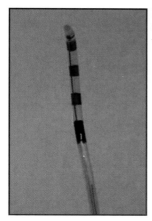

Figure 33-2. Shaping the papillotome wire so that it stays on the left side of the catheter may allow the wire to stay in a more neutral position when traction is applied.

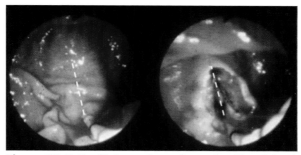

Figure 33-3. Papillotomy is performed with minimal traction on the wire and mild tension to maintain contact of the cutting wire with the tissue. The cut is performed along the "perfect" axis in a stepwise manner.

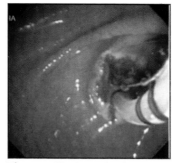

Figure 33-4. Relaxing the papillotome wire allows it to move back to a more neutral position and allows the cutting to be performed along the "perfect" axis.

Control of the Papillotome Wire During Papillotomy

A proper papillotomy requires adequate contact of the cutting wire with the papilla, with sufficient tension on the tissue to allow the wire to cut through the tissue when electrocautery is applied (Figures 33-3 and 33-4). This is achieved by gentle lifting with the elevator, upward angulation of the scope tip, as well as traction on the cutting wire. Torquing the tip of the scope with left wrist movement serves to pull the wire toward a more neutral position. Excess tension or lifting should be avoided because this tends to compress the tissue, making it more difficult to cut, or when excess tension and stretching is applied to the tissue, predisposing to an uncontrolled or zipper cut. Thus, excess tension on the wire, too much lifting with the elevator, and excess tip movement all tend to increase the risk of bleeding and perforation.

Wire-Guided Papillotomy

The use of a hydrophilic-coated wire to stabilize the papillotome during cutting is now routine practice. The guidewire serves to maintain the position of the papillotome in the bile duct and allows a more stable and controlled cut. Minimum traction and gentle lifting of the cutting wire against the tissue (papilla) avoid an excessive cut and its complications.

The Cutting Current

In general, most endoscopists would use a blended (coagulation and cutting) current for papillotomy. To avoid the potential risk of postpapillotomy pancreatitis, some endoscopists suggest that the use of a pure cut current minimizes the risk of coagulation injury around the pancreatic orifice and a lower risk of postpapillotomy pancreatitis.

The amount of wire in contact with tissue will also affect the cut, and that needs to be adjusted accordingly. The usual recommendation is to cut with only one-third of the wire inside the papilla. Too little wire in contact and thus insufficient tension on the tissue may result in only coagulation and an ineffective cut. On the other hand, too much wire inside the papilla may result in an initial inability (failure) to cut and then a zipper cut.

Control Over the Papillotome

Effective papillotomy can be determined by objective assessment of the position of the wire and orientation of the cut from the beginning to the end of the cut. The position of the wire can be changed by manipulating the scope using the up/down and sideways controls. In addition, lifting with the elevator and torquing the scope will place the wire in the desired position. It would help if one maintains a mental picture of the "perfect" axis while performing the papillotomy.

References

1. Leung JW. Fundamentals of ERCP. In: Cotton P, Leung JW, eds. *Advanced Digestive Endoscopy—ERCP.* Boston, MA: Blackwell Publishing; 2005.
2. Leung JW, Leung FW. Papillotomy Performance Scoring Scale: a pilot validation study focused on the cut axis. *Aliment Pharmac Ther.* 2006;24:308-312.

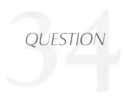
Whenever I Place a Stent for a Stone Impacted Bile Duct or for Bile Leak, the Stent Always Seems to Shift Position Distally. Should I Use a Shorter Stent or a Pigtail Stent? Is There a Trick to Keep These Stents in Place?

Joseph Leung, MD, FRCP, FACP, FACG, FASGE

Stents were first introduced for the management of malignant biliary obstruction. Over the years, we have seen the application of stenting for patients with stone obstruction and acute cholangitis. Stenting for drainage has been used for the management of patients with bile leak to divert the flow back into the duodenum. More recently, prolonged stenting with multiple stents has been recommended for the treatment of benign bile duct stricture.

The design of the stents in general serves two functions: 1) to provide drainage and 2) to prevent migration. In the context of stone disease, stenting also serves the function of preventing stone impaction at the papilla (or papillotomy). Studies have been done to show that for the same caliber, a straight stent with flaps provides much better drainage than a double pigtail stent because of the difference in the size of the side holes (which are much bigger for straight stents). The drainage ability is important when we consider the thick puss-like bile in patients with suppurative cholangitis, which may block the small side holes of pigtail stents. This is the very reason why I advocate the use of larger (10 French [Fr]) straight biliary stents. The same argument can be applied when stents are used for bile leaks (ie, to divert the bile flow to promote healing of the leakage).

The risk of stent migration will depend on the obstructing factor, the size of the common bile duct, and if additional procedures have been performed. Some of the currently available straight stents have a long, straight shaft and an angled distal end; this particular design may not conform to the shape of the bile duct, which varies among patients. If the stent is made of stiff materials, it would tend to migrate to a position that offers least resistance when the tip of the stent is pushing against the wall of the bile duct. Unfortunately, the long, straight shaft of the stent favors downward migration because there is more room in the duodenum to accommodate the distal tip (Figure 34-1).

The second factor is the tightness caused by the impacted stones. If this is a conglomerate of small stones that impact the bile duct, they may provide sufficient friction and resistance to hold the stent in place, but if these stones loosen as a result of a papillotomy and attempted stone extraction, the grip on the stent may decrease and may predispose to stent movement and migration. This is different in the presence of a large stone impacted in the common duct where the stent is being pushed against the bile duct wall (Figure 34-2). The pressure on the stent (which offers resistance to migration) will remain for as long as the stone(s) are intact. The stent may be more prone to migration if it is placed inside a large bile duct following lithotripsy where the stone(s) are broken. Therefore, an additional mechanism is required to prevent stent migration.

If a stent is placed for a stone in the bile duct where there is no stone impaction, the chance of stone and stent movement is high, which may predispose to stent migration. The proximal and distal side flaps on a straight stent serve to prevent stent migration (more so in patients with a bile duct stricture). In the presence of a large papillotomy, upward migration of the stent has been reported. The use of a double pigtail stent may resist stent migration and duodenal injury if the stent does migrate downwards because of the distal pigtail. The proximal pigtail tends to hold the stent inside the bile duct if there is room for the pigtail to reform. The distal pigtail, which usually reforms after stent deployment, will minimize the risk of duodenal injury. However, the double pigtail stents have very small side holes and, for reasons discussed previously, may not provide adequate drainage without a prior papillotomy. We may lose the benefit of drainage. Also, insertion of a double pigtail stent is technically more difficult.

In general, I prefer to use the larger 10-Fr straight stent (Cotton-Leung stent, Cook Medical, Winston-Salem, NC) for biliary drainage, either for bile duct stricture or bile leakage. I use the same stent for managing patients with acute cholangitis and common bile duct (CBD) stone(s). If stents are used for biliary drainage without a defined stricture, I use a 7- to 9-cm stent (depending on the size of the patient) because this will put the proximal tip of the stent into the common hepatic duct area. I do not use shorter stents unless it is for a very distal bile duct stricture. My preference is also to use stents made of polyethylene (because they are softer) rather than the stiffer polyurethane or Teflon (DuPont, Wilmington, DE) because of the ability to shape the polyethylene stents using hot water. The idea of shaping the stent (if necessary) is to create a sufficient (more or less) curvature on the shaft of the stent so that it conforms to the shape of the bile duct when it is in place. At the same time, we can open up the anchoring flaps so that they help to prevent stent migration. The curvature on the mid-shaft of the stent provides a springlike action and helps anchor the stent inside the bile duct. A long, straight shaft is less effective in resisting migration. However, it is not customary for physicians to shape the stents, and therefore, choosing an appropriate design would be of importance.

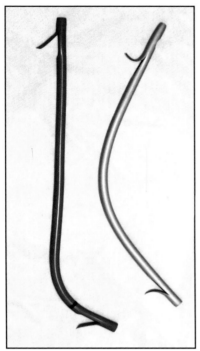

Figure 34-1. Two straight stents with different configurations. The curved stent tends to resist migration.

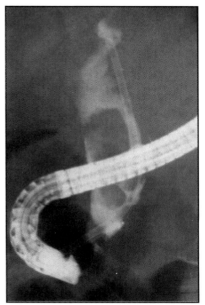

Figure 34-2. Stent for large CBD stone.

It has been reported that up to 30% of large stones will disintegrate spontaneously in the presence of an indwelling stent possibly due to the frictional effect of the stent against the stone or a change in the bile composition as a result of improved bile flow. If the stone becomes smaller, there is an increased chance of stent migration unless the stent has a self-retaining or resistant mechanism against stent migration. In any case, unless the patient is very sick and has a lot of clinical comorbidities, an elective endoscopic retrograde cholangiopancreatography (ERCP) for stent and stone removal should be considered sooner instead of waiting the usual 3 months for stent exchange, as recommended for bile duct strictures. There are other effective modalities for removal of large stones, such as mechanical lithotripsy and intraductal lithotripsy to help ductal clearance, so stenting should only be considered as a temporizing measure. For sick and high-risk patients, long-term stenting has been reported as a definitive treatment for patients with large common duct stones.

It is important to note that the indwelling stent can become blocked with time because of infection, and if a papillotomy has not been done, the patient is at risk of recurrent cholangitis due to stent blockage. These patients should be followed closely and considered for elective ERCP to remove the stone and stent when their clinical condition improves.

SECTION IV

ENDOSCOPIC
ULTRASONOGRAPHY

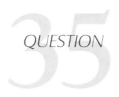
Do All Pancreatic Cysts Need EUS Imaging, and Do They All Need to Be Aspirated for Analysis? Are There Even Standard Criterion to Determine Their Origins?

Christopher J. DiMaio, MD, and William R. Brugge, MD

Pancreatic cystic lesions often present a dilemma to the clinician. These lesions are being discovered more frequently due to the rise in use of cross-sectional imaging for evaluation of other disease processes. A minority of these lesions will present with symptoms. The main concern upon finding any pancreatic cystic lesion is whether or not a malignancy is present and, thus, further investigation is often warranted. However, debate remains on the appropriate evaluation algorithm. Endoscopic ultrasound (EUS) offers high-resolution imaging of cystic lesions and is able to direct fine needle aspiration (FNA) for cytology and cyst fluid analysis. EUS may play a critical role in the evaluation algorithm.

There is a wide differential diagnosis of pancreatic cystic lesions. Lesions can fall into one of three categories: 1) benign, 2) premalignant, and 3) malignant (Table 35-1).

Upon discovering a pancreatic cystic lesion, the evaluation should focus on differentiating between benign and malignant cysts as well as mucinous and nonmucinous cysts.

Before any further imaging or invasive procedures are contemplated, a detailed personal and family history should be obtained from the patient because often clues to the etiology of the lesion may be evident. For example, patients with a history of von Hippel-Lindau disease are at risk for developing serous cystadenomas as well as cystic neuroendocrine tumors. Individuals with an inherited genetic mutation, such as that seen in breast cancer type 2 susceptibility protein (BRCA2) or familial atypical multiple

---

Table 35-1

Types of Pancreatic Cystic Lesions

Benign	Pseudocyst Serous cystadenoma Lymphoepithelial cyst Solid pseudopapillary tumor
Premalignant	Benign mucinous cystic neoplasm (MCN) Intraductal papillary mucinous neoplasm (IPMN)—main duct or side branch
Malignant	Malignant MCN Malignant IPMN—main duct or side branch Cystic degeneration of adenocarcinoma Cystic neuroendocrine neoplasms

---

mole/melanoma (FAMM) syndrome, are at risk for the development of pancreatic cancer. Pseudocysts are common in patients who have had a history of pancreatitis. Though, it must be cautioned that some cystic lesions, particularly if they cause pancreatic duct obstruction, can lead to pancreatitis. A review of a patient's available imaging studies prior to the onset of pancreatitis can be thus be critical.

In addition to a diagnostic evaluation, the patient's symptoms should be assessed for possible linkage with the cystic lesion. A patient who presents with symptoms of abdominal pain and is found to have a pancreatic cystic lesion can be referred directly to surgery, provided the patient is an appropriate surgical candidate. On the other hand, an elderly patient with an incidental, asymptomatic lesion found on computed tomography (CT) imaging will likely benefit from a more detailed evaluation.

Radiologic characteristics of lesions found on standard CT or magnetic resonance imaging (MRI) can also assist in discerning the type of lesion and if malignancy is present. Serous cystadenomas are characterized as having multiple, small, thin-walled cysts in a honeycomb-like pattern. The presence of a central scar on radiologic imaging is often thought of as being pathognomonic of these lesions. Mucinous cystic neoplasms, on the other hand, are oligocystic lesions, with larger cystic compartments, that are typically located in the tail of the pancreas. Radiologic assessment of a lesion's relation to the pancreatic duct can also help in the diagnostic evaluation. Serous cystadenomas and mucinous cystic neoplasms do not communicate with the pancreatic duct, while IPMNs, as their name implies, involve the pancreatic duct. Finally, the presence of an associated mass, invasion of adjacent organs or vasculature, and/or the presence of lymphadenopathy are all suggestive of a malignant pancreatic lesion.

Unfortunately, the utility of cross-sectional imaging in detecting pancreatic cystic lesions is not well matched by its ability to determine the type of lesion. Considerable variability exists in the CT appearance of serous and mucinous pancreatic lesions, and there can be poor interobserver agreement on studies, thus making CT an insensitive tool at distinguishing these lesions.[1] EUS, on the other hand, is extremely useful in providing a detailed analysis of cyst characteristics, particularly in identifying features of malig-

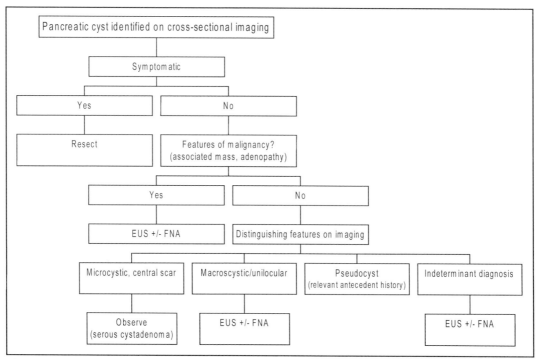

Figure 35-1. Decision algorithm for when to perform EUS ± FNA on pancreatic cysts.

nancy such as wall thickness, macroseptations, intramural nodules or masses, or cystic dilation of the main pancreatic duct.[2] Furthermore, FNA of cystic lesions under EUS guidance allows for the collection of fluid and tissue samples for further analysis. Mucinous lesions (ie, MCNs and IPMNs) characteristically contain thick, viscous fluid as compared to serous lesions that have watery fluid. Cyst fluid is also rich in numerous glycoproteins, many of which can serve as tumor markers. A large prospective study demonstrated that a cyst fluid carcinoembryonic antigen (CEA) level greater than 192 ng/ml was the most accurate test, when compared to EUS alone or cytology, in differentiating mucinous from nonmucinous lesions.[3] Amylase levels also provide information regarding whether a lesion may have communication with the pancreatic duct and would thus be expectedly elevated in IPMNs and pseudocysts. Cytological analysis can provide direct evidence of the presence of malignancy. DNA analysis of cyst fluid for the detection of K-ras and tumor suppressor gene mutations is an emerging modality being used to identify malignant and even premalignant lesions when cytologic material is scant.[4] Perhaps the most powerful aspect of FNA is that it is an extremely safe procedure. In a retrospective review of over 600 patients having undergone EUS with FNA in our center, 13 complications were encountered (2.2%), including 6 patients with pancreatitis (1%).[5] Furthermore, cyst fluid analysis can be performed on as little as 1 ml of fluid for amylase and tumor marker analysis, and only 0.4 ml is required for genetic analysis.

The decision to perform EUS-FNA of a pancreatic cystic lesion is often influenced by clinical factors and radiologic findings, but ultimately it is the concern that a malignancy exists that leads to its performance (Figure 35-1). There is no consensus on the management of premalignant lesions or indeterminate lesions.

Conclusion

Not all pancreatic cysts need EUS imaging or aspiration. However, most lesions are asymptomatic and incidentally found with no relevant antecedent medical history. Furthermore, limitations exist with current cross-sectional imaging in terms of determining cyst type and presence of malignancy. EUS is a proven, safe modality that can provide a high level of detail as well as an opportunity to obtain fluid and tissue samples for a more definitive diagnosis in patients with a pancreatic cystic lesion. Thus, it is our practice to perform EUS with FNA in patients in whom a diagnostic uncertainty exists and where management options would thus be altered.

References

1. Curry CA, Eng J, Horton KM, et al. CT of primary cystic pancreatic neoplasms: can CT be used for patient triage and treatment? *Am J Roentgenol.* 2000;175:99-103.
2. Sedlack R, Affi A, Vazquez-Sequeiros E, et al. Utility of EUS in evaluation of cystic pancreatic lesions. *Gastrointest Endosc.* 2002;56:543-547.
3. Brugge WR, Lewandrowski K, Lee-Lewandrowski E, et al. Diagnosis of pancreatic cystic neoplasms: a report of the cooperative pancreatic cyst study. *Gastroenterology.* 2004;126:1330-1336.
4. Khalid A, McGrath KM, Zahid M, et al. The role of pancreatic cyst fluid molecular analysis in predicting cyst pathology. *Clin Gastroenterol Hepatol.* 2005;3:967-973.
5. Lee LS, Saltzman JR, Bounds BC, et al. EUS-guided fine needle aspiration of pancreatic cysts: a retrospective analysis of complications and their predictors. *Clin Gastroenterol Hepatol.* 2005;3(3):231-236.

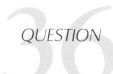
I Am Frustrated by Our Endosonographer Who Frequently Detects Vague Hypoechoic Pancreatic Lesions but Does Not Perform FNA. He Always Recommends Follow-Up EUS in 3 Months. How Often and How Many Follow-Up Examinations Are Needed? Is It Unsafe to Do FNA of the Pancreas?

Kenneth J. Chang, MD, FACG, FASGE

First, it is important to describe what a vague hypoechoic lesion of the pancreas means to an endosonographer (Figure 36-1). Any lesion that is large, well circumscribed cystic, or distorts surrounding structures (main or branch ducts, vessels, etc) does not fall into this category. The differential diagnosis of a vague hypoechoic lesion of the pancreas includes normal changes; chronic pancreatitis (including focal); lobularity (normal parenchyma surrounded by fibrous band); and much less likely a neuroendocrine tumor, lymphoma, metastatic tumor, or early cancer. The two main factors to consider in managing these vague hypoechoic lesions of the pancreas found on endoscopic ultrasound (EUS) are the pretest probability of a neoplastic lesions and the risk of the fine needle aspiration (FNA) itself.

Figure 36-1. EUS image showing a "vague" 5.4 x 5.1 mm hypoechoic lesion in a patient with strong family history of pancreatic cancer.

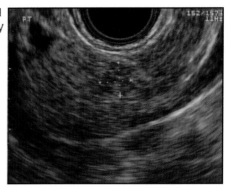

Let us first consider the risk of EUS-guided FNA. In 1996, I reported my early experience among four centers in the United States and Europe. The complication rate for FNA of the pancreas was 2% (among 164 patients), including two major (perforation, bleeding) and two minor (fever) complications.[1] Most recently, a prospective single center study following 355 consecutive patients reported a similar complication rate of 2.5% (95% CI 1.17 to 4.76).[2] Acute pancreatitis occurred in 3 of 355 (0.85%, 95% CI 0.17 to 2.45). None of the patients experienced clinically significant hemorrhage, perforation, or death. In my experience, the risk of pancreatitis is close to 0% when performing FNA into an obvious pancreatic tumor, and I do not hesitate in making multiple passes to secure a tissue diagnosis. On the other hand, I think twice before passing a needle through normal parenchyma or into a vague lesion with a low clinical suspicion. In this scenario, the risk of pancreatitis in my opinion is higher, and the yield of FNA is much lower.

This brings us to consider the pretest probability of a neoplastic lesion. If the pancreas is being examined as part of a routine EUS exam (nonpancreatic indication) and a vague hypoechoic lesion is detected, I would most likely not perform FNA. The only follow-up I would consider would be a repeat EUS in 6 months. In this setting, 3 months is probably too soon to repeat the EUS. If this vague lesion remains unchanged at 6 months, I would not repeat imaging unless clinical symptoms or risk factors change. Other imaging modalities, such as computed tomography (CT) or magnetic resonance (MR) imaging in this setting would most likely not detect an abnormality.

If, however, the indication for EUS of the pancreas is based on relevant symptoms (weight loss, diarrhea, pancreatic-type pain, hypoglycemia, hyperinsulinism, hypergastrinemia, etc) where the pretest probability is higher for a clinically significant lesion, I would be more enthusiastic to perform a EUS-guided FNA. I would try to minimize the number of FNA (1 to 2 passes) and have "real time" dialogue with my cytopathologist in between passes. If the FNA was nondiagnostic, I would repeat an EUS with possible FNA in 3 months. If it is negative again, I would increase the next interval to 6 months (no FNA unless the lesion increases in size).

Finally, you need to consider the special case of a patient with a strong family history of pancreatic cancer. Individuals who have two or more first-degree relatives with pancreatic cancer have a lifetime risk of approximately 16% of developing pancreatic cancer. This is even higher among patients with Peutz-Jeghers or Hereditary Pancreatitis. In these high-risk individuals, a vague hypoechoic lesion in the pancreas has a completely different meaning. These changes may indicate precancerous changes,[3] such as pancreatic

Table 36-1

Management of Vague Hypoechoic Lesion on Pancreatic EUS

Pretest Probability of Neoplastic Lesion	Enthusiasm for Performing EUS-guided FNA	Recommended Surveillance
Low	Low	Repeat EUS in 6 months If no change, no further tests
Medium-high	High	Repeat EUS in 3 months If no change, increase interval to 6 months, etc
Familial pancreatic cancer	High	Consider partial pancreatectomy; otherwise repeat EUS every 6 months

intraepithelial neoplasms (Pan-IN) or intraductal papillary mucinous neoplasm (IPMN) and one should proceed with FNA and consider partial pancreatectomy. If surgery is not performed, close surveillance with EUS (every 6 months) is indicated.

In conclusion, as summarized in Table 36-1, the indication for FNA and the necessity/ timing of repeat EUS in patients found to have vague hypoechoic lesions in the pancreas depend on the clinical scenario (pretest probability).

References

1. Chang KJ, Wiersema M, Giovannini M, et al. Multi-center collaborative study on endoscopic ultrasound (EUS) guided fine needle aspiration (FNA) of the pancreas. *Gastrointest Endosc.* 1996;43:A507.
2. Eloubeidi MA, Tamhane A, Varadarajulu S, Wilcox CM. Frequency of major complications after EUS-guided FNA of solid pancreatic masses: a prospective evaluation. *Gastrointest Endosc.* 2006;63(4):622-629.
3. Canto MI, Goggins M, Yeo CJ, et al. Screening for pancreatic neoplasia in high-risk individuals: an EUS-based approach. *Clin Gastroenterol Hepatol.* 2004;2(7):606-621.

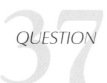
When Is EUS Necessary for a Newly Diagnosed Cancer of the Esophagus, Stomach, Colon, or Pancreas?

Thomas J. Savides, MD

Gastrointestinal (GI) endoscopic ultrasound (EUS) is an important tool for cancer staging because many treatment algorithms are determined by EUS tumor staging. Computed tomography (CT) scan should generally be obtained before EUS to determine if there is any metastatic disease that would make the patient a nonsurgical candidate. If there is no evidence of metastatic disease, then EUS should be performed for loco-regional staging. The tumor-node-metastases (TNM) staging system is used for luminal GI and pancreatic cancer. The EUS accuracy for staging GI and pancreatic cancer is approximately 85% for T-staging and 75% for N-staging. EUS-guided fine needle aspiration (EUS FNA) can be used to obtain tissue diagnosis of tumors as well as peritumoral metastatic disease.

The time to use EUS in cancer staging is before the patient receives any chemoradiation. Staging accuracy significantly decreases after chemoradiation because EUS cannot distinguish between peritumoral inflammation/edema and the actual tumor.

Esophageal Cancer

If EUS shows that a tumor is limited to the mucosal layer (Tis) and without any adjacent lymph nodes (N0), then it is potentially amenable to endoscopic resection. Endoscopic mucosal resection is the only accurate way to know for certain if the tumor is limited to the mucosal layer. Esophageal tumors that invade into the submucosal layer have an approximate 15% risk of metastatic disease to regional lymph nodes and should generally undergo surgical resection with lymph node dissection.

Figure 37-1. Gastric mucosa-associated lymphoid tissue (MALT) lymphoma. Note the thickening of the mucosal and submucosal layers.

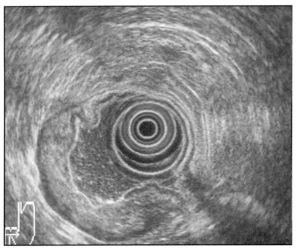

If EUS reveals there is invasion into the periesophageal fat (T3) or periesophageal regional lymph nodes (N1), then the patient is generally referred for preoperative chemoradiation. Patients with involvement into adjacent organs such as the aorta, heart, or trachea (T4) are usually not considered surgical candidates. I do not perform EUS restaging after chemoradiation because it is not accurate and there is no established algorithm for treatment management.

EUS FNA can be performed to increase the lymph node staging accuracy in esophageal cancer.[1] However, often this is not possible due to the lymph nodes being located in a position whereby the needle would need to pass through the tumor to reach the lymph node.

Gastric Cancer

The utility of EUS is limited to evaluating superficial cancer to see if potentially amenable to endoscopic resection. Patients with tumors limited to the mucosa/submucosa (T1) and without adjacent lymph nodes (N0) are candidates for endoscopic resection. For more advanced tumors, there is no need for EUS as these patients will generally go for surgical resection. Occasionally, it may be worthwhile to do an EUS in advanced tumors to determine if there is invasion into an adjacent organ, such as the pancreas. In the rare cases of gastric MALT lymphoma, EUS can identify the tumors limited to the mucosa/submucosa, which are most likely to possibly respond to antibiotic therapy for *Helicobacter pylori* infection (Figure 37-1).[2]

Colorectal Cancer

EUS is only useful in rectal cancer and not helpful in colon cancer.[3] This is because for colon cancer, the surgeon can obtain wide distal, proximal, and lateral margins. In contrast, the location of rectal cancer in the pelvis precludes extended longitudinal or

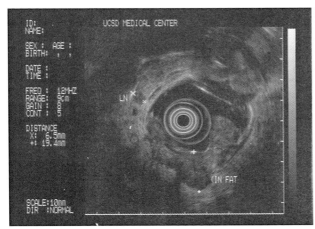

Figure 37-2. Rectal Cancer – Stage T3, N1. Note that the tumor extends into the peri-rectal fat (T3), and there is a malignant appearing lymph node adjacent to the mass (N1).

circumferential surgical margins, which results in a higher risk of locally recurrent tumor after resection. Additionally, because of the fixed position of the rectum in the pelvis, rectal cancer is amenable to radiation therapy.

If EUS shows that the rectal tumor involves only the mucosa/submucosa (T1, N0), then it is amenable to surgical transanal resection. If the tumor extends into the perirectal fat (T3) and/or has associated malignant-appearing lymph nodes (N1), then generally patients are offered preoperative chemoradiation (Figure 37-2). EUS is not routinely performed after chemoradiation for rectal cancer. If a patient undergoes transanal resection of a rectal cancer, then I perform follow-up transrectal ultrasound every 6 months for a total of 2 years to look for any local recurrence.

Pancreatic Cancer

The utility of EUS is somewhat less important for staging pancreatic cancer than esophageal or rectal cancer. This is because although initially EUS was better than old-generation CT scanners for determining locally advanced pancreatic cancer, more recent multidetector CT scans have similar staging accuracies as EUS.[4] Additionally, there are no agreed upon criteria for locally unresectable pancreatic cancer. Invasion of the portal vein (Figure 37-3), superior mesenteric vein, or superior mesenteric artery is generally considered a contraindication to surgery; however, many experienced pancreatic surgeons can often peel pancreatic tumors off blood vessels and do vascular reconstructions for locally invasive cancer. Therefore, in my center, I usually obtain a pancreatic protocol multidetector CT scan rather than an EUS to determine if there are any absolute contraindications to surgery, such as significant encasement of the celiac artery or superior mesenteric artery. There are some centers where more emphasis is placed on the EUS assessment of vascular involvement, although I suspect that multidetector CT scans and MRI scans will continue to be as good as or better than EUS for predicting respectability. In the end, the only true way to know if a pancreatic tumor is resectable is by attempted surgical resection by an expert pancreatic surgeon.

Figure 37-3. Pancreatic Cancer. Note that the mass involves both the common bile duct (CBD) and portal vein (PV).

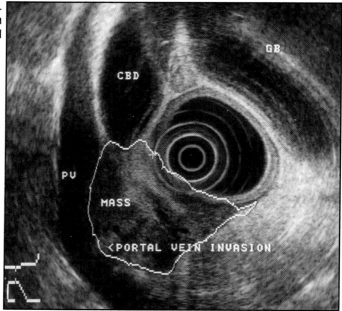

I believe the most important role of EUS in pancreatic cancer is actually visualizing the pancreatic mass (sometimes CT shows only bile duct obstruction or fullness in the pancreatic masses pancreas) and for obtaining FNA cytology tissue diagnosis of malignancy. In the future, EUS-guided fine needle injection may be used for pancreatic cancer treatment either by directly injecting antitumor drugs or by injecting radiopaque markers into the tumor to assist radiation therapy.

References

1. DeWitt J, Devereaux B, Chriswell M, et al. Comparison of endoscopic ultrasonography and multidetector computed tomography for detecting and staging pancreatic cancer. *Ann Intern Med.* 2004;141(10):753-763.
2. Sackmann M, Morgner A, Rudolph B, et al. Regression of gastric MALT lymphoma after eradication of *Helicobacter pylori* is predicted by endosonographic staging. *MALT Lymphoma Study Group. Gastroenterology.* 1997;113(4):1087-1090.
3. Savides TJ, Master SS. EUS in rectal cancer. *Gastrointest Endosc.* 2002;56(4 Suppl):S12-S18.
4. Vazquez-Sequeiros E, Wiersema MJ, Clain JE, et al. Impact of lymph node staging on therapy of esophageal carcinoma. *Gastroenterology.* 2003;125(6):1626-1635.

SECTION V

CAPSULE ENDOSCOPY

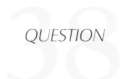
How Do I Manage a Middle-Aged Woman With an Asymptomatic 5-cm, Fluid-Filled Cyst in the Tail of the Pancreas Found Incidentally on Abdominal CT Scanning?

Jacques Van Dam, MD, PhD

The scenario posed in the question above represents a common indication for a visit to my clinic. The increasingly wide-spread use of high-resolution cross-sectional imaging for a variety of indications has led to the now much more common finding of "incidental" abdominal pathology. Asymptomatic patients with incidental findings are managed differently than high-risk patients referred with findings detected in the evaluation of abdominal pain, unexplained weight loss, or other digestive symptoms. The 5-cm cyst described above would be considered large although there is no absolute size below which I would not intervene or above which I would refer for immediate surgical resection. The management of asymptomatic pancreatic cysts is considered controversial as diagnostic tests are considered imperfect and their natural history remains unknown.

As with all clinical assessments, a careful history should be obtained to exclude the possibility of an inflammatory cyst, which is the most common type of pancreatic cyst. A history consistent with acute or chronic pancreatitis, abdominal trauma, or an abnormal hormone-secreting state should be sought and excluded before entering the diagnostic algorithm for cystic neoplasia. A confounding presentation is the patient who suffers an attack of acute pancreatitis due to a complete or partially obstructing cystic neoplasm. In this situation, the pancreatic cyst may be the cause of acute pancreatitis and not the result of it.

One approach to large pancreatic tail lesions in otherwise young healthy patients is to proceed directly to surgery for a distal pancreatectomy. The differential diagnosis for cystic lesions of the pancreas includes malignant and premalignant cystic neoplasms. Because the diagnostic assessment of such lesions with either additional imaging or tissue sampling is not yet perfect, some experts believe that the safest, most conservative approach would be to resect all pancreatic tail pathology in otherwise young healthy patients, including those in whom the lesion was detected incidentally. Distal pancreatectomy is performed for a variety of benign and malignant indications and is associated with far less morbidity and mortality than the Whipple pancreaticoduodenectomy. A retrospective review of the indications and outcomes of distal pancreatectomy from the Johns Hopkins Medical Center was recently reported.[1] The study analyzed the 235 distal pancreatectomies performed between 1994 and 1997. The most common lesion found on distal pancreatectomy was the cystic neoplasm (benign cystadenoma [22%]; cyst adenocarcinoma [3%]) followed by chronic pancreatitis (24%), followed by pancreatic adenocarcinoma (18%) and neuroendocrine tumor (14%). Thus, in this series, the majority of tail lesions resected were benign and malignant neoplasms. Considering that distal pancreatectomy is being performed laparoscopically with increasing frequency, including for "incidentally" detected pancreatic lesions,[2,3] it may be reasonable to limit the diagnostic portion of the management algorithm.

Most recently published reports, however, do not support the resection of all or even most asymptomatic pancreatic cysts. In fact, emerging data suggest that many small asymptomatic cysts lacking "alarm" features may be safely monitored. Allen et al defined a group of patients with pancreatic cysts who may not require resection.[4] In this study of 539 consecutive patients, the investigators concluded that selected patients with cysts less than 3 cm in diameter and without a solid component may be followed radiographically with a risk of malignancy (3%) that is comparable to the risk of mortality from surgical resection. Lahav et al reported on 90 asymptomatic patients (out of 135 who underwent endoscopic ultrasonography for pancreatic cysts) with so-called "indeterminate" or likely mucinous cysts.[5] These patients were followed for a median of 4 years. Malignancy was diagnosed in only one patient after 7 years of follow-up. No patient became symptomatic. Kirkpatrick et al reported that interval cross-sectional imaging with assessment for change or growth of small pancreatic cysts could predict those patients requiring surgery.[6] In this retrospective series of 159 patients' computed tomography (CT) scans with pancreatic cysts, 86 underwent interval imaging performed in less than 6 months (n = 21), 6 to 12 months (n = 22), 1 to 2 years (n = 14), and more than 2 years (n = 29). Solid components recognized in association with the cyst were predictive of malignancy, and pancreatic ductal dilatation was considered a suspicious finding, prompting surgical consideration. The investigators concluded that cystic lesions lacking such radiographic signs could safely be followed by continued imaging.

Does endoscopic ultrasonographic (EUS) imaging have a role in the further characterization of pancreatic cysts? Several studies have assessed the role of EUS to predict the underlying etiology of a cyst based on its size, macro versus microcystic appearance, location in the gland, presence of septae or internal debris, associated solid components, nodules, and thickness of the cyst wall. Predicting malignancy in the early stages of cyst disease remains elusive, however. While some lesions may appear obviously malignant, there are as yet too few endosonographic imaging characteristics to reliably distinguish all benign from premalignant cysts. In addition, the interobserver variation between even experienced endosonographers remains poor.[7] Thus, more definitive data would be required to confidently recommend nonoperative management options.

Modern endosonography includes more than simply imaging. During the past decade, EUS-guided cyst fluid aspiration and analysis has become an important diagnostic adjunct.[8] How to incorporate the data obtained by this minimally-invasive endoscopic procedure into the decision-making process, especially for the asymptomatic patient, remains controversial. One common approach is to divide pancreatic cysts into two groups: 1) those with low risk and 2) those with high risk of current or future cancer. Low-risk cystic lesions include simple cysts, pseudocysts, and serous cystadenomas. High-risk cysts include mucin-producing tumors such as mucinous cystadenomas, mucinous cyst adenocarcinomas, and intraductal papillary mucinous neoplasms (IPMNs) as well as cystic islet cell tumors. There have been several studies evaluating the data for cyst fluid analysis; however, the results are mixed. This led van der Waaij et al to conduct a pooled analysis of previously-published trials.[9] A total of 12 studies were included in the analysis. Cyst fluid chemistries including amylase, CA19-9, and carcino-embryonic antigen (CEA) were evaluated as well as cyst cytology. The authors concluded that cyst fluid analysis was indeed useful in the differential diagnosis of pancreatic cystic neoplasms. Some have found their conclusions too optimistic given a critical review of the data and await a test with improved sensitivity and specificity.[10] As noted above, the current management of pancreatic cysts is controversial.

How then do I manage an asymptomatic woman with an incidentally found cyst in the tail of her pancreas? I obtain a careful and detailed history to exclude a diagnosis of pancreatitis. I obtain a thin-cut, high-resolution, "pancreas protocol" CT scan if not already available and review the CT scan to determine what I can from the appearance of the cyst. If the patient was not referred to me by a surgeon, I typically refer the patient to an experienced pancreatic surgeon for consultation. In my practice, I have discovered that many patients (and some physicians) are not comfortable dealing with the medical uncertainty that a nonoperative treatment plan yields. For such patients, a laparoscopic distal pancreatectomy is a conservative management option. However, recognizing that the risk of malignancy in an incidentally discovered pancreatic cyst in an asymptomatic patient is small (size of 5 cm in the current scenario notwithstanding), I would offer surveillance, in which case an EUS-guided cyst aspiration is an essential part of the initial diagnostic evaluation. I would acquire cyst fluid chemistries, including amylase, CEA, and cyst wall cytology, and manage the patient according to the results, as appropriate.

References

1. Lillemoe KD, Kaushal S, Cameron JL, et al. Distal pancreatectomy: indications and outcomes in 235 patients. *Ann Surg.* 1999;229(5);693-704.
2. Molena D, Primono JA, Khanna A, Schoeniger LO. Laparoscopic distal pancreatectomy is a safe and effective treatment for incidental pancreatic lesions. Abstract: Proceedings of the Society for Surgery of the Alimentary Tract. Los Angeles, CA: 2006.
3. Melotti G, Butturini G, Piccoli M, et al. Laparoscopic distal pancreatectomy: results on a consecutive series of 58 patients. *Ann Surg.* 2007;246:77-82.
4. Allen PJ, D'Angelica M, Gonen M, et al. A selective approach to the resection of cystic lesions of the pancreas: results from 539 consecutive patients. *Ann Surg.* 2006;244:572-582.

5. Lahav M, Maor Y, Avidan B, Novis B, Bar-Meir S. Nonsurgical management of asymptomatic incidental pancreatic cysts. *Clin Gastroenterol Hepatol.* 2007;5:813-817.

6. Kirkpatrick IDC, Desser T, Nino-Murcia M, Jeffrey BR. Small cystic lesions of the pancreas: clinical significance and findings at follow-up. *Abdominal Imaging.* 2007;32:119-125.

7. Ahmad NA, Kochman ML, Brensinger C, et al. Interobserver agreement among endosonographers for the diagnosis of neoplastic versus non-neoplastic pancreatic cystic lesions. *Gastrointest Endosc.* 2003;58:59-64.

8. Rocca R, De Angelis C, Daperno M, et al. Endoscopic ultrasound fine-needle aspiration (EUS-FNA) for pancreatic lesions: effectiveness in clinical practice. *Digest Liver Dis.* 2007;39:768-774.

9. van der Waaij LA, van Dullemen HM, Porte RJ. Cyst fluid analysis in the differential diagnosis of pancreatic cystic lesions: a pooled analysis. *Gastrointest Endosc.* 2005;62:383-389.

10. Pelaez-luna M, Chari ST. Cyst fluid analysis to diagnose pancreatic cystic lesions: an as yet unfulfilled promise. *Gastroenterology.* 2006;130:1007-1009.

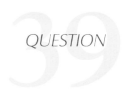
In True Obscure GI Bleeding, What Should I Do if a Capsule Endoscopy and Upper and Lower Endoscopies Are Unrevealing?

Niraj Ajmere, MD, and David Cave, MD, PhD

Identifying the etiology of obscure gastrointestinal (GI) bleeding can be time intensive and frustrating for both clinician and patient. Obscure GI bleeding should be further designated as obscure-overt or obscure-occult before embarking on a diagnostic plan. Obscure-overt bleeding manifests as visible blood (ie, hematochezia or melena) while obscure-occult bleeding may manifest as a positive fecal occult blood test or iron deficiency anemia. This chapter will only consider the former condition.

The first step after negative esophagogastroduodenoscopy (EGD), colonoscopy, and video capsule endoscopy (VCE) is to repeat the colonoscopy and upper endoscopy with or without push enteroscopy. This is particularly true if the patient is referred to you from a source that is not familiar to you. Factors such as the referring endoscopist's experience, different endoscopes with different handling characteristics, and the patient's condition can all affect diagnostic capabilities. The culprit lesion that may have been overlooked at initial EGD and colonoscopy include Cameron's syndrome, ulcers in the duodenal fornices, angioectasias, and Dieulafoy's lesions. The entire VCE should be read by an experienced reader, particularly if the patient is referred.

If the cause of bleeding remains elusive, we would then recommend a repeat VCE to evaluate the small bowel. Two recent studies employing capsules given on the same day[1] and within 4 days of each other[2] noted observer variation of 25% and 27% between the two VCE examinations. This difference in findings is not surprising given the intermittent nature of GI bleeding and the fact that the capsule tumbles. It is likely that only about 70% of the mucosa is seen on any single capsule study. In certain anatomic sites, much less mucosa is seen (eg, the duodenum, where the papilla is seen only a few percent of the time). The data from a second VCE study can aid in planning subsequent therapeutic approaches such as double balloon endoscopy (DBE) or intraoperative enteroscopy.

If a second capsule fails, then DBE can be considered if available. This enteroscope employs the inflation and deflation of two balloons and an overtube for pleating of the small bowel over a 200-cm enteroscope. The entire small bowel can sometimes be examined using a combination of per oral and per rectal approaches although this requires two procedures and cannot be accomplished in all cases. Unfortunately, DBE is not widely available at the present time, is labor intensive, and is technically challenging. The major advantage of DBE over VCE is the potential for therapeutic intervention. A new single balloon enteroscope has recently become available, but there are no comparative data.

A recent series compared the yield of DBE following VCE in 130 patients with obscure GI bleeding. The study reported a DBE miss-rate of 27.8% and a VCE miss-rate of 20.3% for detecting a potential bleeding source. DBE allowed for a variety of interventions, including 35 cases in which argon plasma coagulation or cautery was applied to an arteriovenous malformation (AVM) and 33 cases in which biopsies were taken.[3]

In most cases, we would recommend VCE to identify a treatable lesion prior to undertaking DBE. However, in cases with ongoing obscure-overt bleeding, a decision has to be made as to whether DBE should be performed before VCE given the therapeutic intervention capability of the device or whether to use a technetium bleeding scan followed by angiography and embolization. Angiography will only localize the bleeding lesion if the rate of bleeding is at least 0.5 mL/minute. Angiography can offer therapy with vasopressin infusion or coil embolization. The latter approach is more generally available at present than DBE and is probably safer in the hemodynamically unstable patient since sedation is not needed.

Intraoperative enteroscopy had been used as a method of last resort before the advent of wireless capsule endoscopy for the diagnosis and therapy of obscure GI bleeding. In this procedure, a surgeon sleeves the small bowel over the endoscope while the endoscopist examines the mucosa. While some endoscopists use a per-oral approach, we would advocate introducing the endoscope via a small bowel enterotomy using a sterilized enteroscope sheathed in a plastic sleeve to maintain a sterile operative field. In a large case series published before VCE was widely available, 74% of lesions were identified and treated with intraoperative enteroscopy (IOE).[4] One significant drawback of IOE is mucosal trauma and bleeding caused by pleating of the bowel over the endoscope, thus making differentiation of artifact versus culprit lesions difficult. Also, given the inherent higher risk of IOE complications, including mesenteric tears, perforation, hematoma, infection, and ileus, we would typically recommend IOE in cases where other diagnostic and therapeutic measures had already been attempted and failed.

Small bowel follow-through examination and enteroclysis have very low diagnostic yields for obscure GI bleeding. We do not recommend these tests in the work-up of obscure GI bleeding. However, in cases of suspected small bowel stricturing due to Crohn's disease or non-steroidal anti-inflammatory drugs (NSAIDs) causing possible capsule retention, one should obtain a small bowel follow-through or patency capsule examination prior to VCE.

References

1. Cave DR, Fleisher DE, Gostout CJ, et al. A multi-center randomized comparison of the endocapsule: Olympus Inc and the Pillcam SB: given imaging in patients with obscure GI bleeding. *Gastrointest Endosc.* 2007;65:AB 125.
2. Kimble J, Chak A, Isenberg G, et al. Variation in diagnostic yield back-to-back capsule endoscopy in obscure GI bleeding: final results. *Gastrointest Endoscop.* 2007;65:AB 185.
3. Mehdizadeh S, Ross A, Leighton J, et al. Double balloon enteroscopy (DBE) compared to capsule endoscopy (CE) among patients with obscure gastrointestinal bleeding (OGIB): a multicenter U.S. experience. *Gastrointest Endosc.* 2006;63:AB 91.
4. Kendrick M, Buttar N, Anderson M, et al. Contribution of intraoperative enteroscopy in the management of obscure gastrointestinal bleeding. *J Gastrointest Surg.* 2001;5:162-167.

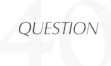

WHAT ARE THE FEATURES THAT DIFFERENTIATE A SUBMUCOSAL BULGE FROM A TRUE MASS ON CAPSULE ENDOSCOPY? WHAT CAN I DO TO CONFIRM A SUBMUCOSAL MASS?

Blair S. Lewis, MD

The proper identification of abnormalities on capsule endoscopy is not an easy task. Unlike standard endoscopy, the capsule reader has to diagnose disease states based on a few images alone. The lesion identified cannot be palpated with biopsy forceps, biopsies cannot be obtained, and a variety of views are often not available. In addition, the images obtained at capsule endoscopy are different from traditional endoscopy since there is no air distention of the bowel wall and the capsule is at times located within millimeters of the mucosa. This is so-called "physiologic endoscopy" where the bowel is not altered by the process of the examination.[1]

The correct diagnosis of a submucosal lesion can be especially difficult since a "bulge" can mimic it. Bulges are indentions of the small bowel wall created by another loop of bowel overlying the loop being inspected. There are visual cues that allow for the differentiation between a bulge and a true mass. Most importantly, one must view the video stream of images and not simply rely on a single image. Bulges from adjacent loops of bowel will peristalse. Peristalsis through the area confirms that the lesion in question is not solid and thus not truly a mass. In addition, inspection of the overlying mucosa can provide clues to differentiate a mass from a bulge. Bulges will have a normal villous pattern over their surface while most submucosal masses will have stretched the mucosa and look thin and translucent (Figures 40-1 and 40-2). A mass lesion can also change the color of the mucosa since, when stretched, the underlying whiteness or grayness of the mass may be apparent.[2] The presence of "bridging folds," valvulae conniventes that stop at the

Figure 40-1. A simple bulge. This fold peristalses with moving images. There is a normal villous pattern.

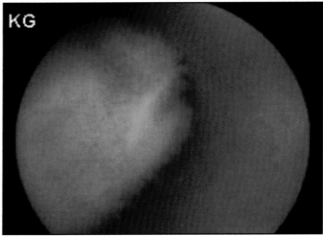

Figure 40-2. A submucosal carcinoid tumor. This does not move with peristalsis and the mucosa overlying is translucent, showing gray tissue beneath.

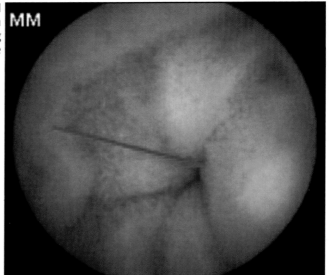

mass's edge and reform on the other side, speaks for a submucosal process. Simple bulges would not make intestinal folds disappear.

At the International Conference on Capsule Endoscopy, a consensus group (Gerard Gay, Warren Selby, Jamie Barkin, C. Fraser, Simon Lo, and E. Toth) proposed to use a series of endoscopic features in an attempt to improve diagnosis of tumors at capsule endoscopy.[3] These are shown in Table 40-1. They were divided into major and minor, and classified into high, intermediate, and low probability.

The following algorithms were developed depending on the probability of a tumor based on Table 40-1. All patients should have cross-sectional imaging with computed tomography (CT), CT enterography, or magnetic resonance imaging (MRI) to assess for extraluminal involvement or metastatic disease. A patient with high or intermediate probability of a tumor needs either double balloon enteroscopy or laparoscopy (Figure 40-3). With a low probability lesion, if no abnormality is seen on CT, then further

Table 40-1

Classification of "Mass" Lesions Seen at Capsule Endoscopy

Major						*Minor*		
Probability of Tumor	Bleeding	Mucosal Disruption	Irregular Surface	Polyploid Appearance	Color	Delayed Passage (≥30')	White Villi	Invagination
High	++	++	++	++	++	++	++	++
Intermediate	+ / –	+	+	+	+			
Low	–	–	–	+ / –	–	–	–	–

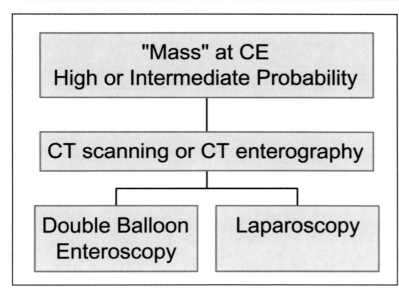

Figure 40-3. Diagnostic algorithm for patients with a high or intermediate probability small bowel (SB) tumor at capsule endoscopy.

management will depend on the clinician's assessment of the significance of the lesion (Figure 40-4).

References

1. Lewis B. Evaluation of capsule endoscopic images. In: Keuchel M, Hagenmuller F, Fleischer D, eds. *Atlas of Video Capsule Endoscopy.* Germany: Springer; 2006:14-23.
2. Lewis B, Keuchel M, Caselitz J. Malignant tumors of the small intestine. In: Keuchel M, Hagenmuller F, Fleischer D, eds. *Atlas of Video Capsule Endoscopy.* Germany: Springer; 2006:172-190.
3. Mergener K, Ponchon T, Gralnek I, et al. Literature review and recommendations for clinical application of small bowel capsule endoscopy—based on a panel discussion by international experts. *Endoscopy.* 2007;39(10):895-909.

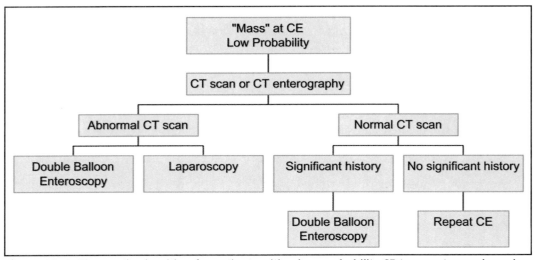

Figure 40-4. Diagnostic algorithm for patients with a low probability SB tumor at capsule endoscopy.

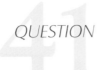
WHAT IS A RELIABLE METHOD TO ESTIMATE THE LOCATION OF A LESION FOUND ON CAPSULE ENDOSCOPY? WHAT IS YOUR APPROACH IF YOU SUSPECT A SUBMUCOSAL MASS BUT ARE NOT CERTAIN WHERE IT IS IN THE SMALL INTESTINE?

Lucinda A. Harris, MS, MD, and Jonathan A. Leighton, MD

Eureka! You found it—the small bowel lesion that caused the obscure gastrointestinal (GI) bleeding or the small bowel tumor responsible for the patient's abdominal pain—it is a great feeling! But wait a minute. "Where exactly in the 600 cm of small bowel is that finding?" you ask as you stare at the monitor looking at a white dot in a sea of squiggles that represent the capsule's course through the small bowel. It looks like it is possibly on the left side to the left of the umbilicus in the left upper quadrant—is that the third portion of the duodenum, or the jejunum, or maybe it is in the colon? At that moment, figuring out exactly where that small bowel lesion is could be a bit overwhelming. However, locating the lesion is so essential to planning the next step in the diagnostic work-up, particularly in localizing occult GI bleeding or in helping the surgeon. For instance, in the case of an arteriovenous malformation (AVM), you would like to localize the lesion to decide if push enteroscopy is all that is needed or whether it is more distal, requiring antegrade double balloon enteroscopy (DBE) to reach and treat the lesion. Additionally, if the AVM is in the distal small bowel, retrograde DBE may be required. When tumors or Crohn's disease strictures are found, then localization is important for surgical intervention or for determining medical therapy.

Figure 41-1. Sensor location guide. (Reprinted with permission from Given Imaging, Ltd.)

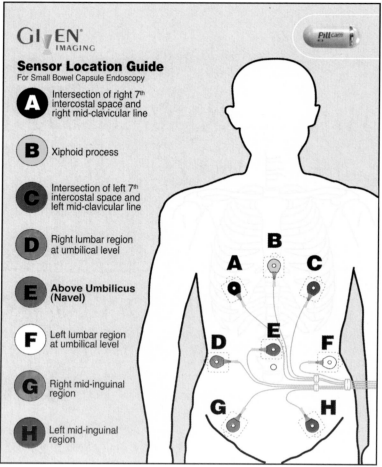

Localization of lesions identified by wireless capsule endoscopy (WCE) can be extremely difficult. Nevertheless, there are several methods for estimating localization of a lesion. What helps us determine where a capsule is in the GI tract? Two features can be very important—anatomic landmarks and keeping track of the elapsed transit time with relation to viewing the landmarks. Certainly, lesions that are close to the duodenal bulb or close to the ileum and the ileocecal valve are most easy to locate. Generally, lesions seen within 30 to 60 minutes of the pylorus are usually able to be seen by push enteroscopy or antegrade DBE.[1,2] Likewise, if the lesion is seen just prior to the capsule entering the ileocecal valve, it will be reachable by retrograde DBE or possibly by colonoscopy.

As the capsule progresses through the small bowel and when the anatomic landmarks are not so clear, it is necessary to rely on the software of the WCE called "the localization module."[3] The capsule software does have a localization method built into the software. To understand this, it is important to understand the sensor array system. A sensor array is applied to the patient's abdomen (eight antennae taped to the belly in a predetermined distribution [Figure 41-1]) that picks up signals from the capsule and carries it to the recording device. The camera chip in the capsule obtains two images/second and transmits its data via radiofrequency to a recording device.[4] The recorder, equipped with a bat-

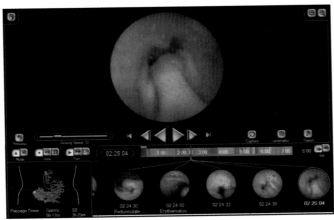

Figure 41-2. RAPID main screen picture of image of a small bowel polyp with the localization figure in the lower left hand corner. (Reprinted with permission from Given Imaging, Ltd.)

tery pack, is then placed in a belt around the patient's waist. The patient can go about his or her daily activities and return in 8 hours so that the sensor array and recording device can be removed. Signals (about 57, 000 images) are then downloaded to the workstation and ready for physician interpretation.

The localization module assists physicians in locating the physical findings identified by the capsule. The strength of the signal emitted by the capsule and received by the eight antennae on the surface of the abdomen helps in determining the true localization of the visible finding. A graphic trajectory of the capsule as it passes through the gastrointestinal (GI) tract is calculated from the output of the localization module and appears in the lower left hand corner of your reading software (Figure 41-2). The module, in calculations reminiscent of college calculus, calculates and presents GI transit times based on the labeled transit times of certain anatomical features (eg, entrance into the stomach, pylorus and passage in into the ileocecal valve, as well as the strength of the radio-frequency [RF] signal). The image data and the levels of the signals received from the sensor array are recorded together. The sensors are arranged in a predefined manner (see Figure 41-1), and the theory of localization is that the closest sensor receives the strongest signal and the location is determined relative to the umbilicus as well as using the sensors with the three strongest signals to triangulate the position of the capsule over the abdominal wall and determine into which of the four quadrants the capsule is located. Figure 41-2 demonstrates a RAPID (reviewing and processing image date) main screen with the image of the finding plus the localization feature in the lower left hand corner. The localization process is a two-dimensional (2-D) estimated location of the capsule based also on the time. As the various anatomic landmarks are seen and captured by the reader, the color of the line on the figure changes. Also the thumbnail feature of capturing the image allows one to label the apparent location of the finding. In the given RAPID imaging system, the stomach is light blue, the small intestine is blue, and the colon is green.

Although the localization module has limitations for individuals in who the capsule remains too long in the stomach/pylorus, the studies have demonstrated that accuracy of this software is variable. Initially, the software was tested by studying normal volunteers. In a study that compared measurements on 17 healthy volunteers (at least four repetitions of capturing capsule images in each individual), the localization calculation was compared with the location of the capsule on fluoroscopic image.[5] Both calculations were made relative to the umbilicus. At least 62% of the calculations were within 4 cm or better of the fluoroscopic image. The cumulative percentage of better than 6-cm accuracy was 87%, and only 5% of the samples were at a significantly higher distance than predicted by the localization module. Another study in 75 patients with a variety of small bowel lesions (predominantly obscure GI bleeding, but also Crohn's disease and other miscellaneous lesions) also verified the accuracy of the localization software.[6] Souquet et al compared an upright abdominal x-ray localization at 2 hours postswallowing the capsule with the localization algorithm.[6] In this case, there was 65% agreement between the radiograph and the automatic device for the localization of the capsule. The most common discrepancy in 18 patients was that, on the localization software, the capsule appeared to be in a lower position than on the abdominal x-ray. Yet another study verified that the capsule was useful at determining whether DBE should be performed and what approach would be most fruitful (oral versus transanal).[7] In this study, 160 patients undergoing WCE primarily for obscure GI bleeding were reviewed, and 38 patients were identified who might benefit from DBE. To determine if an antegrade or retrograde approach would be best, an index of location was devised. This was defined as the time of the capsule to reach the lesions divided by the time of the capsule to reach the cecum. Any individual with a cutoff of value of ≤ 0.75 was thought to require an antegrade approach. Using this approach, the lesions detected by the capsule were reached by DBE in all but two cases, giving a positive predictive value of almost 95% for capsule to discriminate between patients requiring an anal or an oral procedure. Follow-up of these patients at 9 months demonstrated that DBE had positively influenced the management of greater than 90% of the patients.

As outlined previously, accuracy of the current localization algorithm is generally good when combined with time measurements and identification of landmarks, but enhancements are needed. Further advances are being tested in a capsule that incorporates a small magnet and creates a static magnetic field. This model also uses 3-axis sensors, which allow for a better three-dimensional (3-D), rather than 2-D localization.[8] These systems are still in the development phase but will probably allow for improved accuracy in localization of the lesions found on capsule endoscopy.

References

1. Lewis BS. The utility of capsule endoscopy in obscure gastrointestinal bleeding. *Tech Gastrointest Endosc.* 2003;5:115-120.
2. Qureshi WA, Willingham F, Anand B. Localizing the lesion by capsule endoscopy: newer techniques in improving accuracy. *Am J Gastroentero.* 2004;99:S67.
3. Fischer D, Schreiber R, Levi D, Eliakim R. Capsule endoscopy: the localization system. *Gastrointest Endosc Clin N Amer.* 2004;14:25-31.
4. Given Imaging, Expanding the scope of GI. Frequently Asked Questions. Given Imaging Ltd. http://www.givenimaging.com. Accessed November 11, 2007.
5. Costamgna G, Shah SK, Riccioni ME, Foschia F, et al. A prospective trial comparing small bowel radiographs and video capsule endoscopy for suspected small bowel disease. *Gastroenterol.* 2002;123:999-1005.
6. Souquet JC, Bellecose S, Belbouab S, et al. Prospective evaluation of the automatic localization system of the video capsule during small intestine exploration. *ICCE.* 2005;118(Abstract):237.
7. Gay G, Delvaux M, Fassler I. Outcome of capsule endoscopy in determining indication and route for push-and-pull enteroscopy. *Endoscopy.* 2006;38:49-58.
8. Hu C, Meng HQ-H, Mandal M. Efficient linear algorithm for magnetic localization and orientation in capsule endoscopy. IEEE Engineering in Medicine and Biology Society. *Conference.* 2005;7:7143-7146.

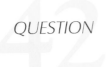

WHEN SHOULD I LOOK FOR POSSIBLE RETAINED ENDOSCOPIC CAPSULES? WHAT SHOULD I DO WHEN THAT HAPPENS?

Lucinda A. Harris, MS, MD, and Jonathan A. Leighton, MD

The expression "an ounce of prevention is worth a pound of cure" applies very well to wireless capsule endoscopy (WCE) and the issue of capsule retention. The first step in avoiding the risk of having a retained capsule is ordering the test for the appropriate indications in patients without contraindications. Indications for WCE are broadening as the technology advances, but generally WCE is indicated for diagnosing obscure gastrointestinal (GI) bleeding, suspected small bowel disease, including Crohn's disease, as well as detecting Barrett's esophagus and esophageal varices. It may also be of benefit in the evaluation of familial polyposis and celiac disease.

Possible contraindications to WCE that might lead to capsule retention include suspected or known small bowel obstruction or stricture, which can be seen with Crohn's disease, nonsteroidal anti-inflammatory drug (NSAID) enteropathy, radiation enteritis, tumor, and a prior surgical anastomosis. To minimize the risk of capsule retention in the small bowel, a careful history should be taken regarding any obstructive symptoms. In these situations, it may be best to noninvasively image the small bowel prior to WCE, especially if the patient is not a surgical candidate. In addition to possible small bowel retention, clinical vignettes have demonstrated the need to take a careful history with regard to swallowing because capsules have gotten lodged in Zenker's diverticulum[1] and at the cricopharyngeus.[2] Additionally, patients who present with symptoms suggestive of a motility disorder—bloating, nausea, or abdominal distention and/or aspiration risk—may not be ideal candidates for WCE or may require endoscopic placement of the capsule.

What does it mean to say a capsule is retained? Interestingly, a formal definition of "retained endoscopic capsules" was not addressed until 2005. At that time, the working group of the International Committee on Capsule Endoscopy (ICCE) agreed to define capsule retention as "having a capsule remain in the digestive tract for a minimum of 2 weeks."[3] They further agreed that a retained capsule would be one that was likely to remain in the bowel lumen unless medical, endoscopic, or surgical interventions were to take place.[3] The committee felt that retention was not to be confused with regional transit abnormalities (RTAs) and defined two different types of RTAs. Type 1 was defined as a capsule remaining in a single segment of the bowel for at least 60 minutes *without* visualization of a mucosal abnormality. A Type 2 RTA was a capsule remaining in a single segment of the bowel for at least 60 minutes *with* the visualization of a mucosal abnormality. Therefore, delayed expulsion (greater than 1 week) not requiring endoscopic or surgical intervention is *not* capsule retention.

The frequency of capsule retention varies with the indication for performing the exam. In general, less than 1% of patients have capsule retention that results in surgery.[4] Several series have looked at capsule retention when performed for different indications such as obscure GI bleeding, previous anastomotic stricture, and/or Crohn's disease and found a range of retention from 6% (occult bleeding) to 21% (in patients with known Crohn's stenosis).[3,5-7]

Until recently, the only way to evaluate the small bowel radiologically consisted of the barium small bowel follow-through or, less commonly, enteroclysis. Despite these diverse methods, the vast majority of retained capsules occurred in patients with normal small bowel radiologic studies,[8] demonstrating that radiologic studies are unreliable in predicting the risk for retention. There are several approaches one can use prior to capsule endoscopy if the concern for retention is significant.

The first approach is to use the new patency capsule. Given Imaging (Duluth, GA) devised a nonradiologic device to evaluate small bowel patency: the Given Patency System.[9] The "patency" capsule (PC) is an inert, self-dissolving capsule (26 mm in length and 11 mm in diameter) that disintegrates after 40 to 100 hours in the gut. The walls of the capsule are made of cellophane filled with lactose mixed with barium, which makes it radiopaque. The capsule surrounds a passive radio-frequency identification tag (RFID). This can be detected by a hand-held radio-frequency scanner or seen on x-ray. There are plugs on either side of the capsule that dissolve slowly and allow entrance of GI fluids into the body of the capsule after 30 to 60 hours. When fluids enter into the body of the capsule, it will dissolve in approximately 10 hours. If there is no obstruction and the pill is excreted intact, this suggests that the intestinal tract is patent. If the scanner or fluoroscopy does not detect the RFID tag at or before 30 hours after ingestion, that would also suggest patency. This has proven to be a very effective tool. Patients that passed the PC intact and without symptoms have successfully undergone WCE.[9]

In addition to the patency capsule, there are radiologic and endoscopic options that can be considered prior to capsule endoscopy if retention is a concern. For those patients who are at risk of having strictures or who are poor operative candidates, one can consider either computed tomography (CT) or magnetic resonance (MR) enterography to aid in evaluating the small bowel and identifying any potential risks of retention. CT and MR enterography can evaluate wall thickness and detect strictures or increased enhancement due to tumor or inflammation and, hence, can be useful in the diagnosis of small-bowel lesions. These techniques have also proven useful to identify extraintestinal abdominal lesions that may aid both in diagnosis and staging of disease. Additionally, double balloon enteroscopy (DBE) is a new endoscopic technique that allows for an extensive evaluation of the small bowel. It can be performed orally or rectally, and in a significant number of cases, a complete small bowel evaluation can be achieved. Larger scale studies are needed to determine the yield and exact role of DBE in patients with occult GI bleeding (OGIB), but DBE appears to be complementary to CE for patients who have OGIB.

Endoscopic placement of the capsule is advised in those patients with dysphagia, risk of capsule aspiration, or suspected/known gastroparesis. The capsule should be placed directly into the small bowel. This can be easily done by front loading the capsule on a gastroscope using a retrieval net, snare, basket, or capsule delivery device. In addition, the patient should be counseled to avoid medications like narcotics, phenothiazines, anticholinergics, or other meds that slow GI motility. With regard to the use of various promotility drugs, study results are mixed.[4] Tegaserod (Novartis, Basel, Switzerland) may have a role in patients who have had slow transit, but the fact that this medication is in marketing and production suspension currently precludes its use.

Once the capsule is ingested, it is necessary to make certain that the capsule has been excreted. The majority of patients will witness excretion of the capsule. If the patient does not observe passage of the capsule or the capsule does not reach the colon, then capsule excretion should be confirmed. It is easier to diagnose retention when there is clear visualization of an obstructing lesion but trickier to identify when there is excessive luminal debris. Sometimes one has the feeling of "déjà vu" when the same mucosal areas are repetitively seen. Unfortunately, colonic nonvisualization cannot be used as an absolute indicator since up to 25% of capsule examinations fail to enter the colon during the 8 hours of data acquisition and this may only indicate slowed transit.[3] If the capsule reaches the colon, it is not necessary to document excretion.

If a retained capsule is a concern, an abdominal x-ray is the single best diagnostic modality for ruling out this possibility. Other radiologic modalities—barium enema, abdominal and pelvic CT scan, and small bowel series—may be helpful in more precise localization. The exact timing of when to obtain an abdominal film for suspected retention is at the physician's discretion but is usually done after 2 weeks.[10] There are also certain mitigating circumstances influencing timing of the x-ray. These reasons include the patient's need for reassurance, presence of obstructive symptoms, and a study done in a patient with a known contraindication or the patient who needs to undergo an MRI.

If capsule retention is diagnosed, then either endoscopic or surgical intervention may be indicated. Fortunately, most cases of capsule retention remain asymptomatic and acute obstruction is rare. Although the data is scant, medical therapy with steroids or biologic therapy may be tried in the case of Crohn's disease with strictures. In suspected NSAID enteropathy, it would be reasonable to stop the medication and observe. Lavage solutions have occasionally been effective but have to be used cautiously. However, no successful data on medical therapies per se (steroids, prokinetics, laxatives, infliximab, stopping NSAIDs) have been reported to aid the capsule in passing. If the patient has no obstructive symptoms and slow transit is suspected, it may be reasonable to delay intervention. The capsule literature does describe a case of a patient with celiac disease who had delayed transit in a more involved area of the jejunum and eventually passed the capsule.[11] Endoscopic retrieval has been reported[12,13] and can take place using traditional endoscopy, colonoscopy, or DBE depending on the capsule's location. Although surgical intervention is to be avoided unless absolutely necessary, several case reports have highlighted that the operation not only removed the capsule but also was therapeutic—identifying and relieving the obstruction.[14-16]

In summary, once an accurate history has screened out patients with known contraindications, a retained capsule becomes a relatively rare occurrence. However, patients at higher risk of retention remain those individuals with stricturing small bowel disease, particularly those with Crohn's disease. This patient population may derive special benefit from screening modalities such as CT and MR enterography and/or the PC. Once retention is suspected an abdominal x-ray is the single best means for detection of the capsule. Endoscopy, particularly DBE, has evolving roles in retrieving a capsule, and the role of medical therapy is still evolving. Although a last resort in capsule retention, surgery has proven useful in some individuals for both diagnosing the underlying disorder as well as retrieving the capsule.

References

1. Geller, AJ. Video capsule impaction in a Zenker's diverticulum: letters to the Editor. *J Clin Gastroenterol.* 2005;39:647-648.
2. Fleischer DE, Height RI, Nguyen CC, et al. Videocapsule impaction at the cricopharyngeus: a first report of this complication and its successful resolution. *Gastrointest Endosc.* 2003;57:427-428.
3. Cave D, Legnani P, de Franchis R, Lewis BS. ICCE consensus for capsule retention. *Endoscopy.* 2005;37:1065-1067.
4. Vanderveldt HS, Barkin JS. Capsule endoscopy: a primer for the endoscopist: Ten ways to prevent capsule retention and delayed passage. *Tech Gastrointest Endos.* 2006;8:164-168.
5. Barkin JS, Freindman S. Wireless endscopy requiring surgical intervention; the world's experience. *Am J Gastroenterol.* 2002;97:S298.
6. Sears DM, Avots-Avotins A, Clup K, Gavin M. Frequency and clinical outcome of capsule retention during capsule endoscopy for GI bleeding of obscure origin. *Gastrointest Endosc.* 2004;60:822-827.
7. Cheifetz A, Sachar D, Lewis B. Small bowel obstruction: indication or contraindication for capsule endoscopy. *Gastrointestin Endosc.* 2004;59:AB461.
8. Barkin JS, O'Loughlin C. Capsule endoscopy contraindications: complication and how to avoid recurrence. *Gastrointest Endosc Clin N Am.* 2004;14:61-65.
9. Signorelli C, Rondonotti E, Villa F, et al. Use of the Given Patency system for the screening of patients at high risk for capsule retention. *Digestive Liver Dis.* 2006;38:326-330.
10. Sachdev MS, Leighton JA, Heigh RI, et al. A prospective study of the utility of abdominal X-ray post capsule endoscopy for the diagnosis of capsule retention. *Gastrointest Endosc.* 2007;66(5):894-900.
11. Guerrero R, Lara LF, Browning JD. A case of diarrhea, ataxia and capsule endoscopic retention. *Dig Dis Sci.* 2007;52(11):3174-3177.
12. Arifuddin RM, Baichi MM, Mantry PS. Small bowel capsule impaction and successful endoscopic retrieval. *Clin Gastroent Hepatol.* 2005;3(1):A34.
13. Tanaka S, Mitsui K, Shirakawa K, et al. Successful retrieval of video capsule endoscopy retained at ileal stenosis of Crohn's disease using double-balloon endoscopy. *J Gastroenterol Hepatol.* 2006;21(5):922-923.
14. Gonzalez Carro P. Intestinal perforation due to retained wireless capsule endoscope. *Endoscopy.* 2005;37:684.
15. Fry LC, de Petris G, Swain JM, Fleischer DE. Impaction and fracture of a video capsule in the small bowel requiring laparotomy for removal of the capsule fragments. *Endoscopy.* 2005;37:674-676.
16. Strosberg J, Shibata D, Kvols LK. Intermittent bowel obstruction due to a retained wireless capsule endoscope in a patient with small bowel carcinoid tumour. *Can J Gastroenterol.* 2007;21:113-115.

SECTION VI

MISCELLANEOUS

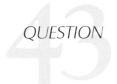

If I Suspect a Small Bowel Lesion, How Do I Choose Among Small Bowel Series, Capsule Endoscopy, CT Enterography, and Double Balloon Enteroscopy as the Diagnostic Test?

Hendrikus S. Vanderveldt, MD, MBA, and
Jamie S. Barkin, MD, FACP, MACG, AGAF, FASGE

The classic approach to a patient with a suspected small bowel lesion has been to use radiological imaging as an initial diagnostic choice. However, recent advances in endoscopic technologies have provided a wider range of choices. Each test or procedure, however, has its own availabilities, limitations, benefits, and drawbacks; therefore, the appropriate diagnostic choice should depend on both the suspected problem as well as the resources available to the clinician.

A common choice in initial diagnostic imaging is the small bowel series (SBS). It is widely available and easy to perform. However, as the orally ingested contrast is primarily designed to create a radiological mucosal relief pattern, its diagnostic usefulness is limited to large endoluminal growths or irregularities. Patients in whom large masses or cancers, strictures, or ulcerations are suspected are the best candidates for this study. Even in this group, the overall diagnostic yield of SBS is low, and therefore, a negative study does not rule out the possibility that a lesion or stricture might still exist. For example, a recent meta analysis comparing the yield of SBS to capsule endoscopy for nonstricturing small bowel Crohn's disease found that SBS had a diagnostic yield of only 23%.[1]

Other radiological choices for small bowel imaging include computed tomography enterography (CTE). CTE uses both a neutral oral contrast and intravenous contrast to create cross-sectional images of the abdomen, highlighting the small bowel. CTE provides excellent views of the mucosa of the small bowel, the bowel wall, as well as the adjacent organs. In addition, CTE's capability for multiphasic imaging also allows the radiologist to evaluate vascular anomalies. Consequently, CTE can be used both in patients with suspected endoluminal masses as well as those with suspected vascular anomalies such as arterio-venous malformations. The diagnostic capabilities CTE were shown to be much better compared to SBS. In addition, when CTE was compared to ileos-copy, sensitivity and specificity in detecting active inflammation of the terminal ileum in patients with Crohn's was 81% and 70%, respectively.[2] However, CTE is not without its drawbacks. First, its availability is usually limited to tertiary centers. Second, CTE is costly and involves significant radiation exposure to the patient. Last, CTE may not be a consideration in patients with iodine allergies or in whom vascular access is unavail-able.

The endoscopic procedures for evaluating small bowel lesions include both wireless capsule endoscopy (WCE) and double balloon enterography (DBE). WCE is a relatively noninvasive procedure that provides direct mucosal visualization of the small bowel. Therefore, it is useful in evaluating endoluminal lesions, vascular anomalies, as well as subtle mucosal changes such as villous blunting. Although relatively new, WCE is now widely available. Overall, for a diagnostic small bowel mucosal or endoluminal evalua-tion, WCE provides a superior yield to both traditional imaging and push enteroscopy. Thus, we feel that WCE is the gold standard in evaluating the patient with a suspected mucosal small bowel lesion. Numerous studies have been conducted that support this assertion but perhaps the most interesting are those that compare the diagnostic yields of different tests in the investigation of patients with obscure gastrointestinal (GI) bleed-ing. These are most interesting because the causative problem or source in obscure small bowel gastrointestinal bleeding can vary widely, covering the gamut of small intestinal diseases from neoplastic masses to vascular malformations. As a result, when discussing the diagnosis of small intestinal disease a clinician can use the overall yield in obscure GI bleeding as a rough "yardstick" to evaluate the overall effectiveness of that test for a wide spectrum of small bowel diseases.

Triester et al performed a meta-analysis of diagnostic procedures for obscure GI bleed-ing using 20 different studies involving over 500 patients.[3] They found that WCE was superior to both push enteroscopy and small bowel barium radiography for diagnosing significant small intestinal disease. The incremental yield or IY (defined as the yield of WCE minus the yield of the comparative modality) of WCE over push enteroscopy and small bowel radiography was greater than or equal to 30% for each. Interestingly, the Triester article also included studies that compared WCE to nontraditional imaging modalities such as CTE, mesenteric angiogram, and small bowel magnetic resonance imaging (MRI) (one study for each different modality).[3] Of these, only the study involv-ing small bowel MRI rose to the level of statistical significance and in that one study WCE was again found to be superior (IY = 36%).

WCE is not always the best test when evaluating or diagnosing small bowel disease. The major drawback to using this modality is that it does not offer a therapeutic option at the time of the procedure. Another potential drawback is capsule retention. Although the overall rate of capsule retention is low (around 1%),[4] capsule retention has never occurred in the absence of an organic structural narrowing. Consequently, a retained capsule can provide useful information about the location of the pathological process. This informa-tion can then direct a therapeutic modality (ie, DBE or interoperative enteroscopy).

DBE is a direct endoscopic evaluation that has the potential of visualizing the entire small bowel. It involves sequentially inflating one or two separate balloons on an endoscope to allow the physician to telescope the small bowel over the scope, thereby advancing the enteroscope through the small bowel. Overall, the rate complication has been noted to be around 1.7% (0.8% in diagnostic studies/4.3% in therapeutic studies).[5] Its availability, however, is limited and it is an expensive and lengthy procedure often lasting up to three hours. Therefore, DBE is best viewed in the context of being utilized to follow up a positive finding discovered during an initial test.

In conclusion, our choice of modality, either radiological or endoscopic for diagnosing small bowel lesions depends on our clinical suspicion as to the type of lesion. Radiological studies should be considered more strongly when there exists a concern for large potentially obstructing lesions or when extraluminal manifestations of disease are suspected. Endoscopic studies should be considered when the direct visualization of the mucosa is desired or if a therapeutic option is needed. Additionally, as disease processes evolve over time and no test has a perfect diagnostic capability, some patients may require multiple diagnostic modalities in order to properly diagnose their underlying problem.

References

1. Triester S, Leighton JA, Leonitiadis GI, et al. A meta-analysis of the yield of capsule endoscopy compared to other diagnostic modalities in patients with non-stricturing small bowel Crohn's disease. *Am J Gastroenterol.* 2006;101:954-964.
2. Bodily KD, Fletcher JG, Solem CA, et al. Crohn disease: mural attenuation and thickness at contrast-enhanced CT enterography—correlation with endoscopic and histologic findings of inflammation. *Radiology.* 2006;238:505-516.
3. Triester S, Leighton JA, Leonitiadis GI, et al. A meta-analysis of the yield of capsule endoscopy compared to other diagnostic modalities in patients with obscure gastrointestinal bleeding. *Am J Gastroenterol.* 2005;100:2407-2418.
4. Vanderveldt HS, Barkin JS. Capsule endoscopy: a primer for the endoscopist: ten ways to prevent capsule retention and delayed passage. *Tech Gastrointest Endosc.* 2006;8:164-168.
5. Mensink PB, Haringsma J, Kucharzik T, et al. Complications of double balloon enteroscopy: a multicenter survey. *Endoscopy.* 2007;39(7):613-615.

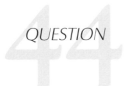

What Is the Proper Way of Performing an Intraoperative Enteroscopy, and When Should It Be Done in Place of the Other Nonoperative Ways of Examining the Small Intestine?

Blair S. Lewis, MD

Capsule endoscopy has rapidly become the third test in the evaluation of patients with obscure gastrointestinal (GI) bleeding and is considered the state-of-the-art method for visualizing the small intestinal mucosa.[1] Lesions identified at capsule endoscopy often require therapeutic intervention, including cauterization of bleeding vascular lesions or excision of neoplasms. Push enteroscopy is limited in its depth of insertion and even 2.5-meter long enteroscopes can only reach the proximal jejunum. Double balloon enteroscopy (DBE) allows for deeper intubation and this procedure cannot only be performed from the standard peroral route but can also be advanced into the small bowel in a retrograde manner from a peranal approach.[2] American experience with DBE has shown that this technique, even when performed from both the oral and transrectal approaches, does not view the entire small bowel.[3] DBE is not routinely available. Despite this latest technology, total intubation of the small bowel cannot be achieved in every patient, and thus, not every small bowel lesion is amenable to nonsurgical therapy.

After capsule endoscopy, intraoperative enteroscopy remains the most common form of total small bowel endoscopic examination. Colonoscopes are routinely employed for this examination, though a push enteroscope may also be used. The instrument does not need to be sterile since the recommended technique involves peroral intubation of the small intestine. The proximal jejunum is intubated prior to the performance of the laparotomy since, once the abdomen is open, it may be difficult to advance the

Figure 44-1. The patient is explored laparoscopically.

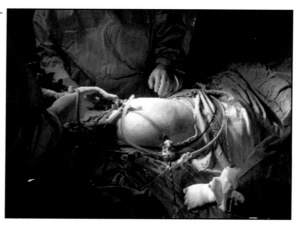

instrument around the ligament of Treitz due to excessive and unopposed bowing of the endoscope shaft along the greater curvature of the stomach. With oral intubation of an adult colonoscope, the endotracheal tube cuff may need to be deflated to permit passage of the wide caliber endoscope. Once the colonoscope is placed within the proximal jejunum, laparotomy is performed. A noncrushing clamp is placed across the ileocecal valve to prevent distention of the colon with insufflated air. Colonic distention can lead to difficulties with subsequent abdominal closure. The endoscopic exam is performed by having the surgeon grasp the endoscope tip and hold a short segment of bowel straight to allow endoscopic inspection. The view is best seen by dimming the overhead lights and allowing the surgeon to look at the transilluminated bowel. Once examined both internally and externally, the small bowel is pleated onto the shaft of the endoscope, and the next section of bowel is examined. Active bleeding within the small bowel may limit the effectiveness of this examination. Generally, examination is performed only during intubation since mucosal trauma occurs with the pleating, causing artifact that may be confused with the appearance of angioectasia.[4] Lesions identified with intraoperative enteroscopy are marked by the surgeon with a suture placed on the serosal surface of the small intestine. At the end of the examination, the endoscope is withdrawn, and sites of resection are identified by the sutures.

There are other techniques of intraoperative enteroscopy. This author performs an enterotomy through which an enteroscope covered by a sterile plastic sheath is placed (Figures 44-1 to 44-5). The site of the enterotomy is generally determined by findings at capsule endoscopy. For example, a distal lesion seen on capsule endoscopy is approached through an enterotomy in the distal small bowel. An enterotomy performed in the mid-small bowel allows for both proximal and distal intestinal intubation. Using an enterotomy allows the exam to be performed in a laparoscopically assisted manner with a much small incision. In addition, the use of CO_2 (CO_2Efficent, E-Z-EM, Lake Success, NY) for insufflation eases wound closure due to its rapid absorption by the mucosa.

Intraoperative endoscopy has been used for several reasons. Intraoperative enteroscopy is presently the endoscopic method most widely used in identifying small intestinal sites of bleeding. This most typically involves the bleeding site identified on capsule endoscopy and not approachable by endoscopic means. Intraoperative enteroscopy is also used in cases in which surgical guidance is needed to limit small bowel resection. This is

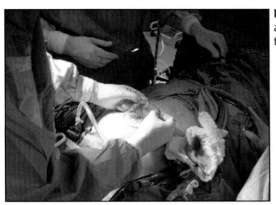

Figure 44-2. The general area identified to be abnormal by capsule endoscopy is exteriorized through a small incision.

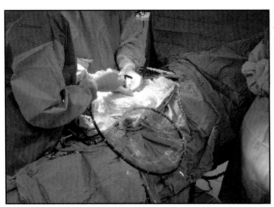

Figure 44-3. A standard enteroscope is passed through a sterile sleeve while an enterotomy has been created in the bowel wall.

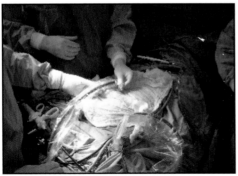

Figure 44-4. Intraoperative enteroscopy is performed in this laparoscopically assisted method.

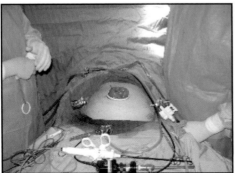

Figure 44-5. Upon completion, the bowel with sutures affixed to the areas of abnormality are seen prior to surgical resection.

especially true in patients with hereditary hemorrhagic telangiectasia (HHT) syndrome where there are often diffuse lesions that are limited to the jejunum. The diffuse nature limits enteroscopic management, and the surgeon needs to know where these lesions cease. Intraoperative enteroscopy is also used in patients with small bowel polyposis such as Peutz-Jeghers syndrome. Multiple polypectomies can be performed, and the specimens can be removed through the enterotomy, limiting resection. Finally, intraoperative enteroscopy has been used to identify and guide resection of diaphragm disease of the small bowel. These stenoses of the small bowel are not palpable, and endoscopic guidance is often necessary intraoperatively.

References

1. Raju G, Gerson L, Das A, Lewis B. American Gastroenterological Association (AGA) Institute Medical Position Statement on Obscure Gastrointestinal Bleeding. *Gastroenterology.* 2007;133(5):1694-1696.
2. Raju G, Gerson L, Das A, Lewis B. American Gastroenterological Association institute technical review on obscure gastrointestinal bleeding. *Gastroenterology.* 2007;133(5):1694-1696.
3. Mehdizadeh S, Ross A, Gerson L, et al. What is the learning curve associated with double balloon enteroscopy? Technical details and early experience in 6 US tertiary care centers. *Gastrointest Endosc.* 2006;64:740-750.
4. Frank M, Brandt L, Boley S. Iatric submucosal hemorrhage: a pitfall of intraoperative endoscopy. *Am J Gastroenterol.* 1981;75:209-210.

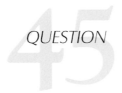
WHAT CAN AN ENDOSCOPIST DO TO EVALUATE UPPER ABDOMINAL PAIN IN PATIENTS WHO HAVE UNDERGONE GASTRIC BYPASS SURGERY FOR OBESITY?

Lynne Do, MD, and Joseph Leung, MD, FRCP, FACP, FACG, FASGE

In the evaluation of abdominal pain in the post gastric bypass patient, a review of the prior surgical history will guide decision making before proceeding with possible upper endoscopy. This can include the type of bariatric surgery and when it was performed.[1] The anatomical details of the procedure should be elucidated either via discussion with the patient's surgeon, a review of the operative reports, or postoperative imaging studies. Various forms of bariatric surgery have been developed over the past 50 years, with the Roux-en-Y gastric bypass (RYGBP) being the most commonly performed in the United States today. The RYGBP typically involves the formation of a small (<30 mL) gastric pouch along the lesser curvature by suture or staples. A small stoma measuring 10 to 12 mm connects the gastric pouch via an end-side anastomosis to the jejunum. The Roux limb can measure 60 to 150 cm with a blind end measuring 1 to 2 cm.

Other types of bariatric surgery include vertical banded gastroplasty, gastric banding, and biliopancreatic diversion with or without duodenal switch. However, we will limit the discussion to the commonly performed surgery in the United States.

The differential diagnosis for abdominal pain can be quite varied depending on the time interval since surgery and the constellation of symptoms as possible hints to the underlying cause. In the early postoperative period, abdominal pain, nausea/vomiting, and bloating may simply be due to poor postgastric bypass diet adherence (ie, overeating or eating too fast), thus emphasizing the importance of good symptoms and dietary history. In such cases, dietary education may need to be re-emphasized with the patient.

However, more serious complications may be the cause of the abdominal pain and nausea in the post gastric bypass patient. Stomal or marginal ulcerations can occur in up to 16% of post gastric bypass patients but usually occur more than 6 to 8 weeks post-operatively.[2] Contributing factors include focal acidity due to staple line dehiscence with gastrogastric fistula, increased gastric pouch size, nonsteroidal anti-inflammatory drugs (NSAIDs), *Helicobacter pylori*, and focal microvascular ischemia at the anastomosis. The ulcerations are often located on the jejunal side of the anastomosis. The diagnosis is best made with endoscopy. Treatment includes proton pump inhibitors (PPI), with or without sucralfate, avoidance of NSAIDs, and evaluation for gastrogastric fistula. If there is excess bile reflux and persisting abdominal pain, one may consider lengthening the Roux limb.[3] These ulcers can also present with gastrointestinal (GI) bleeding, which may require endoscopic therapy with epinephrine injection, thermo or electrocautery, or hemoclipping, as indicated.

Another complication of gastric bypass that can present with abdominal pain and nausea is stomal stenosis. This may be accompanied by gastric pouch dilatation, retained food in the pouch, bezoar, or an anastomotic ulcer. However, if stenosis is seen within days to weeks after surgery, the narrowed stoma may be attributed more to the surgical procedure. Diagnosis can be confirmed on endoscopy or with upper GI barium studies. Treatment consists of surgical revision in those with early symptoms, whereas for those with late postoperative symptoms, PPI are given for marginal ulcers. If ulcer is excluded, the stenosis is dilated with the through-the-scope balloon up to a maximum diameter of 15 mm.

Staple line dehiscence or gastrogastric fistula may also complicate the postoperative course in a gastric bypass patient. This can be heralded by abdominal pain and weight regain. Diagnosis is confirmed with an upper GI series or endoscopy. Endoscopically, the dehiscence may appear somewhat like a diverticulum. During endoscopy, clips may be placed to repair the defect; otherwise, surgical revision may be warranted. There have also been preliminary reports of injection of sclerosants such as sodium morrhuate, fibrin glue, hemoclip, or endoscopic suturing to decrease the size of an enlarged gastric stoma due to staple line dehiscence.[4]

Partial small bowel obstruction should be considered as a source of abdominal pain and nausea/vomiting in any postsurgical patient. Abdominal films, an upper GI series, or computed tomography (CT) scan are useful in the diagnosis. Conservative management, including supportive measures such as bowel decompression and bowel rest may be sufficient. However, some patients may require surgical treatment of the small bowel obstruction.

Lastly, gallstones are a frequent postoperative occurrence with the underlying rapid weight loss. Symptoms include postprandial abdominal pain with nausea/vomiting and occasional jaundice. Evaluation consists of liver function tests, abdominal ultrasound, magnetic resonance cholangiopancreatography (MRCP), and less likely, percutaneous transhepatic cholangiography. In patients status post-RYGBP, evaluation and treatment of underlying hepatobiliary pathology by endoscopic retrograde cholangiopancreatography (ERCP) is more technically demanding. There have been reports of successful ERCPs performed with the assistance of double balloon enteroscopy (DBE) in some centers. Ultimately, cholecystectomy may be indicated.

In summary, the evaluation of abdominal pain in a post gastric bypass patient should take into consideration the details of postoperative anatomy, specific accompanying symptoms, and time interval since surgery.

References

1. Stellato TA, Crouse C, Hallowell PT. Bariatric surgery: creating new challenges for the endoscopist. *Gastrointest Endosc.* 2003;57:86-94.
2. MacLean LD, Rhode BM, Nohr C, Katz S, McLean APH. Stomal ulcer after gastric bypass. *J Am Coll Surg.* 1997;185:1-7.
3. Kaplan LM. Gastrointestinal management of the bariatric surgery patient. *Gastroenterol Clin N Am.* 2005;34:105-125.
4. Huang CS, Farraye FA. Endoscopy in the bariatric surgical patient. *Gastroent Clin N Am.* 2005;34:151-166.

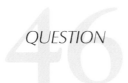

WHAT ARE THE PROVEN SUCCESSFUL ENDOSCOPIC METHODS IN TREATING GASTROINTESTINAL FISTULA?

Fauze Maluf Filho, MD, and Paulo Sakai, MD, PhD, FASGE

A fistula is defined as the presence of an abnormal communication between two organs or between an organ and the cutaneous surface. It can be caused by benign inflammatory diseases (eg, actinic rectovaginal fistula), malignancy (eg, tracheoesophageal fistula), or iatrogenic maneuvers (eg, anastomotic leaks). It is impossible to cover the treatment of all kinds of gastrointestinal (GI) fistula in a few words, but their management follows certain basic principles. Before considering an endoscopic treatment, one must have in mind that there are some general rules that apply for the treatment of GI fistula.

The fistulous tract must be adequately drained. This is particularly true for the external anastomotic leaks. It is common that the draining tube is so far from the GI wall that it causes the formation of an infected fluid collection between the two orifices. When the fluid collection is full, its content is then expelled through the fistulous tract, reaching the drain and the skin. In order to correct this situation, the drain must be advanced through the fistulous tract crossing the collection until it reaches the anastomotic orifice.

The treatment of infection must be optimal. Endoscopic injection of sealing agents such as cyanoacrylate or fibrin glue does not work adequately in infected fistulous tracts.

The nutritional support should be adequate. GI fistulas impose major energy and fluid losses.

GI stenosis, when associated with the fistula, should be adequately managed. This is somewhat common for anastomotic leaks where a stenosis is present. Endoscopic dilation will definitely accelerate the rate of the closure of the fistula. At the same session of endoscopic dilation, surgical materials such as threads and displaced staples should be removed because they can cause foreign body inflammatory reaction. Dealing with a critically ill patient suffering from a postoperative fistula demands a prompt and effective treatment. In those cases, our choice is the placement of a self-expandable plastic stent that should be left in place for 4 weeks. If the fistulous anastomosis in the upper GI tract is wide open, some care should be taken to prevent the distal migration of the stent. We use a thread that is passed through the proximal part of the stent, and it is exposed through the nostril. We have tried to clip the proximal part of the stent to the GI wall, but it has not worked well even when using larger clips. Another option is to place a self-expandable metallic stent with a thread attached to the proximal end of the stent, in the format of a lasso, thus it is possible to remove it (Hanarostent, M.I. Tech Co, Ltd, Seoul, Korea). To avoid migration, there is an alternative; attach a long silk thread to the patient's earlobe.

Malignant fistulas will not seal even when adequate drainage, treatment of infection, and nutritional support are provided. A malignant fistula is a very good indication for a self-expandable metallic or plastic stent. The most common example is malignant tracheoesophageal fistula for which the placement of a covered self-expandable stent will palliate dysphagia and seal the leak in more than 90% of patients.[1]

Even when all the above mentioned principles of GI fistula management are respected, some cases remain unsolved. For those patients, different endoscopic treatments have been tried with heterogeneous results. In our opinion, all of those techniques should be considered as adjuvant treatments for the management of recalcitrant GI fistulas. Endoscopic clipping is an attractive option, but it should be remembered that apposition of mucosal surfaces is not enough for promoting healing. There are reports about small fistulous orifices that were closed by endoscopic clipping. Larger gastrogastric leaks after Roux-en-Y gastric bypass (RYGBP) were successfully managed by burning the edges of the fistula with argon plasma followed by clipping.[2]

There are descriptions of fibrin glue or cyanoacrylate injection in small fistulous tracts along the GI tract. In almost all descriptions, the technique involved some kind of scarification of the fistulous tract before injecting the sealing agent. Occasionally, a combination of techniques is necessary, involving denuding mucosa, clip placement, and gluing.[2] The placement of self-expandable plastic and covered metallic stents has been our choice for the treatment of large fistulous orifices or in critically ill patients with postoperative anastomotic leaks. For small fistulous orifices, we have been using a biomaterial made from porcine small intestinal submucosa. It is a collagen biomatrix that provides a tissue integration, replacing and repairing damaged tissue (SurgiSiS, Cook Surgical, Winston Salem, NC). It has been used for the treatment of inguinal hernia repair, dura mater replacement, lower limb venous ulcers, and anal fistulas. The material is available a sheet and a plug, suitable for endoscopic placement into the fistulous tract (Figure 46-1).

The endoscopic management of GI fistula demands a careful patient selection and close communication with the patient's surgeon. Likely in the near future, the accessories in development for natural orifice translumenal endoscopic surgery (NOTES) will be very useful for closing GI fistulas.

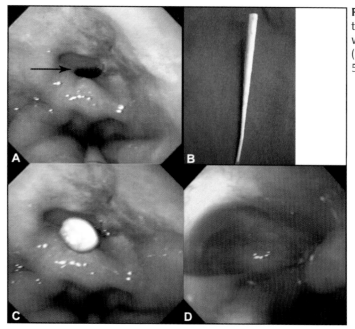

Figure 46-1. Gastrocutaneous fistula after (A) RYGBP being stuffed with (B, C) SurgiSis plug and (D) fistula closure achieved after 5 weeks.

References

1. Ross WA, Alkassab F, Lynch PM, et al. Evolving role of self-expanding metal stents in the treatment of malignant dysphagia and fistulas. *Gastrointest Endosc.* 2007;65:70-76.
2. Merrifield BF, Lautz D, Thompson CC. Endoscopic repair of gastric leaks after Roux-en-Y gastric bypass: a less invasive approach. *Gastrointest Endosc.* 2006;63:710-714.

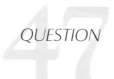

BOUGIENAGE, BALLOON DILATION, CAUTERY CUTTING, STENTING, AND STEROID INJECTION HAVE ALL BEEN DESCRIBED TO TREAT BENIGN STRICTURES. IS THERE A RIGHT WAY OF DOING THIS?

David L. Carr-Locke, MD, FRCP, FASGE

Benign esophageal stricture is not a single animal but more a population of pathologies and etiologies that results in the nonmalignant narrowing of one or more regions of the esophagus, causing dysphagia when the lumen decreases to 12 mm or less. Not surprisingly, therefore, no one therapy is likely to fit all circumstances. I think of the solution to this problem as a range and sequence of therapies. The objective is to restore normal swallowing and maintain it with as few interventions as possible, reducing patient discomfort while limiting the risk of perforation and improving quality of life.

The first step is to define the stricture as accurately as possible and its etiology since this will determine the risk of therapy (eg, compare eosinophilic esophagitis with peptic stricture), likely prognosis, and use of adjunctive treatments such as a proton pump inhibitor, topical steroids, or the need for surgery. Contrast radiology, such as a barium swallow and computerized tomography (CT), may give additional information about stricture extent, motility, and extraesophageal disease. However, endoscopy can provide almost all of the information necessary using the range of endoscopes and sampling devices now available, allowing visualization of the proximal aspect of the stricture, stricture length and appearance, and the state of the esophagus or stomach distal to the stricture. Combination with fluoroscopy is mandated when the stricture can only be traversed by a guidewire, when injection of radiographic contrast through the endoscope is desirable, and when a fistula is suspected and/or stent placement is anticipated. The historical requirement for a pre-endoscopy barium study is no longer applicable.

The second step is dilation therapy, and for the majority of strictures, balloon dilation or bougienage is equally effective. Modern hydrostatic balloons come as wire guided (preloaded or not preloaded) or nonwire-guided (flexible plastic leading tip) versions and bougies as wire-guided or nonwire-guided types.[1] There is little if any reason (except self-dilation) for using the older mercury or equivalent-filled nonwire-guided dilators. Balloons, although more expensive than reusable bougies, have become popular since they are passed through the endoscope and are positioned under direct endoscopic guidance. I will usually gauge the luminal diameter of the stricture by sight and start with a balloon 1 to 2 mm larger than this as the first dilation size, increasing with the same three-stage balloon to 2 or 3 mm larger. If the dilation is easy, without pain or severe mucosal tearing (remember that there is always some), I continue to dilate to as near 18 mm as possible. Obvious perforation or bleeding can be treated immediately by the application of endoscopic clips. The "rule of 3's" no longer strictly applies to balloon dilation but, since perforation is a risk with every dilation no matter how many times it has been accomplished, common sense should prevail when dilating from one diameter to another (eg, 5 to 18 mm may be too much for one session).

If the dilation proves to be difficult to achieve because of elasticity of the stricture (eg, caustic or radiation strictures) or is too painful for the patient, or there is excessive mucosal disruption, consider injecting triamcinalone[2] and/or incising the stricture with a needle knife.[3] I have used these techniques very rarely.

The third step is maintaining a lumen long term, and this has traditionally been achieved by repeated dilation, as dictated by recurrent symptoms. If the interval between dilations is tolerable to the patient and endoscopist (ie, every few months or years), then this strategy is acceptable. The stricture that fails to respond to these standard methods or requires a repeated dilation after short intervals of less than 1 month is often termed *refractory*. Such strictures should be considered empirically for additional methods of treatment such as the steroid injection and cautery incision already mentioned. The newer and more predictable choice, however, is the temporary placement of a removable expandable stent for approximately 6 weeks to allow remodeling of the stricture to the stent diameter, which ranges from 16 to 20 mm. Success rates of 80% should be expected with this strategy.[4]

In summary, you should approach the benign esophageal stricture as a staged sequence of diagnosis, dilation, and assessment of response. Most strictures of all etiologies will respond to simple mechanical dilation with mandatory follow-up and access to the endoscopy team at short notice should symptoms reoccur. Additional therapy will be required for a small percentage of the most difficult strictures, and remember that malignancy can masquerade as a benign stricture at first presentation, especially when there is no clear etiology.

References

1. ASGE Technology Committee. Tools for endoscopic stricture dilation. *Gastrointest Endosc.* 2004;59(7):753-760.
2. Ramage JI Jr, Rumalla A, Baron TH, et al. A prospective, randomized, double-blind, placebo-controlled trial of endoscopic steroid injection therapy for recalcitrant esophageal peptic strictures. *Am J Gastroenterol.* 2005;100(11):2419-2425.
3. DiSario JA, Pedersen PJ, Bichiş-Canoutas C, Alder SC, Fang JC. Incision of recurrent distal esophageal (Schatzki) ring after dilation. *Gastrointest Endosc.* 2002;56(2):244-248.
4. Conigliaro R, Battaglia G, Repici A, et al. Polyflex stents for malignant oesophageal and oesophagogastric stricture: a prospective, multicentric study. *Eur J Gastroenterol Hepatol.* 2007;19(3):195-203.

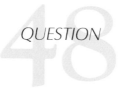

FEWER AND FEWER SIGMOIDOSCOPIES ARE BEING PERFORMED. SHOULD WE EVEN BOTHER DOING THEM?

Thomas M. Zarchy, MD, and Francis A. Farraye, MD, MSc

Since the publication of the multicenter Veterans Administration (VA) cooperative retrospective screening colonoscopy study,[1] there has been a steady decline in the utilization of flexible sigmoidoscopy (FS) in the United States. However, in our era of restrained colonoscopy capacity, FS remains an option for colorectal cancer screening. It has been shown in randomized and case control studies to decrease the incidence of colon cancer.[2,3] It does not require space and staff for recovery and can be performed effectively by physicians' assistants.[4] In experienced hands, FS is extremely safe and only takes about 5 minutes to perform. It causes only mild discomfort when a <10 mm diameter scope (ie, diagnostic upper endoscope) is used.[5] FS is the main method of colorectal cancer screening in England and is still being performed in centers of excellence in the United States.[6,7]

Most of the FS literature involves its use for colon cancer screening. There have been recent references that indicate that the yield of FS for advanced neoplasms (AN) in screening average risk individuals under age 60 approaches the yield of colonoscopy.[8,9] AN are defined as neoplasms ≥1 cm or containing villous histology, high-grade dysplasia, or cancer. They are widely used as surrogate markers for colon cancer. Imperiale et al constructed a validated risk score in asymptomatic patients ≥50 for AN proximal to the splenic flexure.[8] Their scale is based on age, gender, and the histology of polyps found on colonoscopy distal to the splenic flexure. They concluded that FS might be sufficient for the large minority of their patients who were at low risk for AN. In a large multicenter randomized prospective Italian study, colonoscopy had a statistically insignificant 1.08 odds ratio (OR) (0.74 to 1.57) for AN over FS in patients aged 55 to 59 years.[9] On the other hand, colonoscopy demonstrated a statistically significant 2.00 OR (1.30 to 3.09) for AN over FS in patients aged 60 to 64 years.[9] These findings are consistent with those from the retrospective multi-center VA cooperative study (mean age of 63).[1] The advantage of colonoscopy in patients over 60 is related to the increasing proximal distribution of AN in older patients.

Some areas regarding screening FS remain controversial.[6] These include whether patients with 1 or 2 diminutive adenomas require follow-up colonoscopy[6] and the interval between FS. In the United States, intervals of 5 years are generally recommended.[6] In England, they are presently in the midst of a prospective study involving a once in a lifetime screening exam at age 55.[7]

FS has also been useful in surveillance for patients after low anterior resection for rectal cancer because of the high local recurrence rate.[10] Flexible sigmoidoscopy is also used to follow postcolectomy patients with residual rectal tissue and diagnoses of ulcerative colitis or familial adenomatous polyposis.

There is limited literature on the use of FS in symptomatic patients. A recent electronically published study demonstrated that symptoms did not predict an AN proximal to the rectosigmoid but rectal bleeding correlated with an AN in the rectosigmoid.[11] Studies comparing a diagnostic FS to colonoscopy for rectal bleeding have reached conflicting conclusions.[11,12,13] The American Society for Gastrointestinal Endoscopy (ASGE) state in their 2005 Standards of Practice paper, "because most patients with scant hematochezia have an anorectal or a distal colonic source of bleeding, the initial evaluation in young, healthy patients ($\leq$40 years of age) should be a digital rectal examination and sigmoidoscopy with or without anoscopy."[14] They recommend colonoscopy for those over age 50 or with risk factors such as anemia.[14] Evidence-based studies in patients aged 40 to 49 with scant hematochezia would be beneficial.

Flexible sigmoidoscopy is often used as a first line diagnostic tool for acute diarrhea, particularly when left-sided colitis is expected.[15] It can be performed quickly and safely. It is helpful in diagnosing and assessing the severity of ulcerative colitis and pouchitis. In cases of chronic diarrhea, FS can also be useful, but it will miss localized right-sided macroscopic colitis (ie, Crohn's disease, tuberculosis, amebiasis, cytomegalovirus [CMV]) and localized right-sided microscopic colitis. Hence, colonoscopy may be the better choice. In patients with acquired immune deficiency syndrome (AIDs) and diarrhea, FS with biopsy has been recommended by the ASGE as a first-line diagnostic test.[14] Evidence-based studies are needed comparing FS and colonoscopy for chronic diarrhea.[15]

In conclusion, FS remains a valuable tool for colorectal cancer screening and as a diagnostic tool for certain symptomatic patients. It is best considered as synergistic rather than competitive to colonoscopy.

References

1. Lieberman DA, Weiss DG, Bond JH, et al. Use of colonoscopy to screen asymptomatic adults for colorectal cancer. *N Engl J Med.* 2000;343:162-168.
2. Thiis-Evensen E, Hoff GS, Sauer J, et al. Population base surveillance by colonoscopy: effect on the incidence of colorectal cancer. *Scand J Gastroenterol.* 1999;34:414-420.
3. Selby JV, Friedman GD, Quesenberry CP, Weiss NS. A case control study of screening sigmoidoscopy and mortality from colorectal cancer. *N Engl J Med.* 1992;326:653-657.
4. Schoenfeld PS, Cash B, Kita J, et al. Effectiveness and patient satisfaction with screening flexible sigmoidoscopy performed by registered nurses. *Gastrointestinal Endosc.* 1999;49:158-162.

5. Farraye FA, Horton K, Hersey H, et al. Screening flexible sigmoidoscopy using an upper endoscope is better tolerated by women. *Am J Gastroenterol.* 2004;99(6):1074-1080.
6. Levin TR, Farraye FA, Schoen RE, et al. Quality in the technical performance of screening flexible sigmoidoscopy: recommendations of a multi-society international task group. *Gut.* 2005;54:807-813.
7. Atkin WS, Edwards R, Wardle J, et al. Design of a multicentre randomised trial to evaluate flexible sigmoidoscopy in colorectal cancer screening. *J Med Screen.* 2001;8:137-144.
8. Imperiale TF, Wagner DR, Lin CY, et al. Using risk for advanced proximal colonic neoplasia to tailor endoscopic screening for colorectal cancer. *Ann Intern Med.* 2003;139:959-965.
9. Segnan N, Senore C, Andreoni B, et al. Comparing attendance and detection rate of colonoscopy with sigmoidoscopy and FIT for colorectal cancer screening. *Gastroenterology.* 2007;132:2304-2312.
10. Rex DK, Kahl CJ, Levin B, et al. Guidelines for colonoscopy surveillance after cancer resection: a consensus update by the American Cancer Society and the US Multi-Society Task Force on Colorectal Cancer. *Gastroenterology.* 2006;130:1865-1871.
11. Zarchy TM, Tsai F, Ramicone E, Chan LS. A risk profile for advanced proximal neoplasms on diagnostic colonoscopy. *Digest Dis Sci.* 2008, in press.
12. Van Rosendaal GM, Sutherland LR, Verhoef MJ, et al. Defining the role of fiberoptic sigmoidoscopy in the investigation of patients presenting with bright red rectal bleeding. *Am J Gastroenterol.* 2000;95:1184-1187.
13. Lewis JD, Brown A, Locallo R, Schwartz JS. Initial evaluation of rectal bleeding in young persons: a cost effective analysis. *Ann Intern Med.* 2002;136:99-110.
14. Standards of Practice Committee. ASGE Guideline: the role of endoscopy in the patient with lower GI bleeding. *Gastrointest Endosc.* 2005;62:656-659.
15. Standards of Practice Committee. Use of endoscopy in diarrheal illnesses. *Gastrointest Endosc.* 2001;54:821-823.

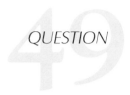
When Should I Perform a Push Enteroscopy, and Are Overtube and Fluoroscopy Necessary for the Procedure?

Christopher J. Gostout, MD

Push enteroscopy remains a useful procedure for both diagnosis and therapy of small intestinal disease, especially disease confined to the proximal small bowel (duodenum and proximal jejunum). The availability of balloon enteroscopy has expanded access into the small bowel from above and below (via the colon) and has not supplanted the value and need for push enteroscopy. As time limits are being imposed on the length of balloon enteroscopy, especially when time limitations encroach upon 1 hour, an important cross-over in techniques and clinical situations then occurs, which creates confusion as to what procedure to perform.

The following are strong indications to perform push enteroscopy:

* Duodenal disease such as suspected neoplasia (idiopathic; Peutz-Jegher's syndrome) or obscure acute bleeding.

* Surveillance for the familial adenomatous polyposis (FAP) syndrome given evidence that significant sized polyps typically drop off beyond the ligament of Treitz.

* Acute bleeding in the presence of an abdominal aortic graft.

* Endoscopic retrograde cholangiopancreatography (ERCP) in postoperative anatomy, Bill Roth II, and Roux-en-Y.

* All gastrointestinal (GI) bleeding of obscure origin.

* Abnormalities seen during capsule endoscopy within 30 minutes of duodenal entry.

* Proximal small bowel obstruction.

* The diagnostic evaluation of upper gastrointestinal (UGI) tract postoperative anatomy.

* Initial efforts at coagulation therapy for known symptomatic small bowel angiodysplasia.

* Direct percutaneous endoscopic jejunostomy (PEJ) placement.

The above indications influence the choice of endoscope needed. There are some rules of thumb that can be applied to help make an instrument selection among an adult colonoscope, pediatric colonoscope, and a push enteroscope. Both a pediatric and an adult colonoscope (insertion tube length 160 cm) will predictably access the small bowel to within 10 to 20 cm of the ligament of Treitz. With effort, these instruments can be passed considerably beyond, as proven by their use for ERCP in the setting of a Roux-en-Y anatomy. The adult colonoscope is of particular value for performing ERCP during which there is a high likelihood of biliary stenting. The adult colonoscope has a therapeutic-sized working channel to allow passage of a 10-French (Fr) stent. The adult colonoscope will also allow convenient placement of a palliative self-expanding metal stent (SEMS) in the setting of malignant obstruction. The pediatric colonoscope is otherwise an excellent choice for most push enteroscopy applications within the very proximal small bowel, in particular the duodenum and for performing a direct PEJ. Formal push enteroscopy with a dedicated enteroscope (insertion tube length 230 to 250 cm) is an unequivocal choice in all patients with obscure GI bleeding and possibly in all patients who have capsule endoscopy abnormalities within the proximal half of the small intestine. My own practice-based cost modeling, in the setting of obscure bleeding, favors push enteroscopy prior to capsule endoscopy.

Push enteroscopy is limited by insertion tube loop formation. Using a colonoscope, this occurs predominantly within the stomach but also within the small bowel. The latter is more prominent when adult colonoscopes are used. Gastric looping can be partially overcome when instruments with a variable stiffness insertion tube are employed. The "stiffening" on these instruments begins at approximately 35 to 40 cm from the tip. Gastric loops can be reduced after which the stiffness is applied. The stiffer insertion tube may create problems with small bowel looping as it is advanced. Straightening and shortening of the small bowel can be achieved by on/off use of the stiffness feature and applying loop reduction maneuvers as in colonoscopy. Push enteroscopy with colonoscopes does not require fluoroscopy. This procedure is similar to performing a colonoscopy in a redundant colon, which is commonplace to perform successfully.

As mentioned above, all cases of obscure occult bleeding deserve push enteroscopy using a formal push enteroscope. This instrument will significantly exceed the depth of insertion obtainable with a colonoscope. It must, however, be used with an overtube if this benefit is to be obtained. Years ago, I assessed depth of insertion comparing a push enteroscope with an overtube versus a pediatric colonoscope via abdominal x-ray documentation. The results were striking. This study also demonstrated that the overtube may not necessarily eliminate the gastric loop when it does not pass beyond the pylorus. Excessive looping hampers using a push enteroscope without an overtube and is not worth the effort. I have had the luxury of using a push enteroscope with variable stiffness to the insertion tube and a therapeutic channel. The insertion tube stiffness feature is set back from the tip 95 to 100 cm. This allows insertion into the small bowel, straightening, stiffening with gastric loop reduction, and the maintenance of desirable flexibility of the forward portion of the insertion tube for navigating small bowel loops and turns. In a formal comparison using a standard overtube, it offered as good a depth of insertion and significantly better than insertion without any overtube. Fluoroscopy is also not necessary, unless used for ERCP, enteral SEMS placement, or there is an ana-tomic/radiologic targeted area for which fluoroscopy will provide feedback as to reaching this site. Fluoroscopy is of little value otherwise other than satisfying one's curiosity or confirming one's frustration.

The success of push enteroscopy with a dedicated instrument and overtube is depen-dent upon patience, allowing sufficient time for the procedure (1 hour), and skill in advancing the overtube. The latter will make or break the procedure. There are basic steps that will enable success. The overtube should be kink-free at all times (during use, repro-cessing, and storage). Both the overtube and the endoscope must be liberally lubricated, especially the inside of the overtube. Once the overtube is passed, lubricating jelly should be continually applied in front of the overtube as it is slid over the enteroscope insertion tube toward the patient. The lubricant will provide a useful leading edge and some will pass between the insertion tube and the overtube, greatly enhancing passage of the over-tube over the endoscope. The overtube should not be advanced until the enteroscope has been passed beyond the duodenal bulb and the insertion tube is straightened, completely reducing the gastric loop. A gastric loop always occurs when the enteroscope is passed through the pylorus and the duodenal bulb. The overtube should be passed until there is resistance, which is typically at the pylorus. At this point, pushing both the endoscope and the overtube simultaneously, gently and slowly, will enable critical passage of the overtube into the duodenum and will minimize the risk of recurrent gastric looping.

There are two clinical settings worth specifically mentioning. First is the patient with known angiodysplasia involving the small intestine. If there are multiple lesions to vary-ing depths, it may be possible to reduce transfusion needs by ablating all those lesions that can be accessed. Before embarking on time consuming and technically more challenging balloon enteroscopy, push enteroscopy with overtube and coagulation therapy should be attempted first. Second is the patient with identified abnormalities seen on capsule endoscopy beyond 30 minutes of duodenal entry. Some of these patients may have their findings reached using push enteroscopy. I have found it practical to look at the capsule localization map to help decide whether or not a push exam with an overtube is worth the attempt. If the abnormality is beyond duodenal entry by three distinguishable loops, then the procedure is unlikely to succeed. If the number of loops cannot be determined, then a cut-off time of 1 hour beyond duodenal entry is used to make the decision.

In summary, push enteroscopy continues to be a mainstay in the evaluation and ther-apy of small intestinal disease and in the postoperative anatomy. It is a technique with a practical value that can be forgotten in the shadow of balloon enteroscopy enthusiasm. Fluoroscopy offers little if any benefit, except when push enteroscopy is performed for ERCP in the postoperative anatomy of a Roux-en-Y or a Bill Roth II or in the placement of an enteral SEMS.

References

1. Harewood G, Gostout CJ, Farrell MA, Knipschield MA. Prospective controlled assessment of variable stiffness enteroscopy. *Gastrointest Endosc.* 2003;58(2):267-271.
2. Gostout CJ, Bender CE. Cholangiopancreatography, sphincterotomy, and common duct stone removal via Roux-en-Y limb enteroscopy. *Gastroenterology.* 1988;95(1):156-163.
3. Singh P, Amitabh C. Push-type enteroscopy in occult gastrointestinal bleeding. *Tech Gastrointest Endosc.* 2003;5(3):109-114.
4. Lichtenstein G. Post-surgical anatomy and ERCP. *Tech Gastrointest Endosc.* 2007;9(2):114-124.
5. Dunkin B, Martinez J. Biliary and pancreatic duct access after bariatric surgery. *Tech Gastrointest Endosc.* 2007;9(3):183-188.
6. Fang J. Percutaneous access for enteral nutrition. *Tech Gastrointest Endosc.* 2007;9(3):176-182.

INDEX

CURBSIDE
Consultation

The exciting and unique *Curbside Consultation Series* is designed to effectively provide gastroenterologists with practical, to the point, evidence based answers to the questions most frequently asked during informal consultations between colleagues.

Each specialized book included in the *Curbside Consultation Series* offers *quick access* to *current* medical information with the ease and convenience of a conversation. Expert consultants who are recognized leaders in their fields provide their advice, preferences, and solutions to 49 of the most frequent clinical dilemmas in gastroenterology.

Written with a similar reader-friendly Q and A format and including images, diagrams, and references, each book in the *Curbside Consultation Series* will serve as a solid, go-to reference for practicing gastroenterologists and residents alike.

The series editor is Francis Farraye, MD, MSc, Clinical Director, Section of Gastroenterology, Boston Medical Center

Titles include:

Curbside Consultation of the Colon: 49 Clinical Questions
Brooks D. Cash, MD, FACP, CDR, MC, USN

Curbside Consultation in Endoscopy: 49 Clinical Questions
Joseph Leung, MD, FRCP, FACP, FACG, FASGE, and Simon Lo, MD

Curbside Consultation in GERD: 49 Clinical Questions
Philip Katz, MD

Curbside Consultation of the Liver: 49 Clinical Questions
Mitchell Shiffman, MD

Curbside Consultation of the Pancreas: 49 Clinical Questions
Scott Tenner, MD, MPH, and Alphonso Brown, MD, MS CLIN Epi

Curbside Consultation in IBD: 49 Clinical Questions
David Rubin, MD; Sonia Friedman, MD; and Francis A. Farraye, MD, MSc

WWW.CURBSIDECONSULTATIONS.COM

Please visit

www.slackbooks.com
to order any of these titles!
24 Hours a Day...7 Days a Week!

Attention Industry Partners!

Whether you are interested in buying multiple copies of a book, chapter reprints, or looking for something new and different—we are able to accommodate your needs.

Multiple Copies

At attractive discounts starting for purchases as low as 25 copies for a single title, SLACK Incorporated will be able to meet all of your needs.

Chapter Reprints

SLACK Incorporated is able to offer the chapters you want in a format that will lead to success. Bound with an attractive cover, use the chapters that are a fit specifically for your company. Available for quantities of 100 or more.

Customize

SLACK Incorporated is able to create a specialized custom version of any of our products specifically for your company.

Please contact the Marketing Communications Director of Health Care Books and Journals for further details on multiple copy purchases, chapter reprints or custom printing at 1-800-257-8290 or 1-856-848-1000.

*Please note all conditions are subject to change.

CODE: 328

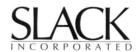

SLACK Incorporated • Health Care Books and Journals
6900 Grove Road • Thorofare, NJ 08086

1-800-257-8290 or 1-856-848-1000

Fax: 1-856-853-5991 • E-mail: orders@slackinc.com • Visit www.slackbooks.com